SKIN CANCER:

A Book That Will Give You A Better Understanding Of What Skin Cancer Is, Its Symptoms, Treatment, Choice of Diet ,Tips On Coping With It And More!

By

George M. Rogers.

COPYRIGHT

TABLE OF CONTENTS

CHAPTER 1

Understanding What Skin Cancer is

Nearly one in five persons acquire skin cancer sometime in their lives. Nearly all skin cancers may be cured if identified and treated early. Treatments include excision, cryotherapy, Mohs surgery, chemotherapy and radiation. Check your skin for any changes in size, shape or color of skin growths. See your dermatologist once a year for a professional skin checkup.

Normally, new skin cells arise as cells get old and die or when they become injured. When this mechanism doesn't operate as it should, a fast increase of cells (some of which may be aberrant cells) follows. This clump of cells may be noncancerous (benign), which doesn't spread or cause damage, or cancerous, which may spread to neighbouring tissue or other locations in your body if not discovered early and treated.

Skin cancer is typically induced by ultraviolet (UV) light exposure from the sun.

THERE ARE THREE MAIN TYPES OF SKIN CANCER:
- Basal cell carcinoma.
- Squamous cell carcinoma.
- Melanoma.

Basal cell carcinoma and squamous cell carcinoma are the most prevalent kinds of skin cancer and are frequently dubbed "non-melanoma skin cancer."

Melanoma is not as prevalent as basal cell or squamous cell carcinomas but is the most severe kind of skin cancer. If left untreated or found at a late stage, melanomas are more likely to spread to organs outside the skin, making them difficult to cure and possibly life-limiting.

Fortunately, if skin cancer is diagnosed and treated early, most are curable. This is why it is crucial to take a few protections and to consult with your healthcare physician if you suspect you have any indicators of skin cancer.

HOW COMMON IS SKIN CANCER?
Skin cancer is the most prevalent cancer diagnosed in the U.S.

OTHER SKIN CANCER FACTS:
- Around 20% of Americans develop skin cancer sometime in their life.
- Approximately 9,500 Americans are diagnosed with skin cancer every day.
- Having five or more sunburns throughout your life increases your likelihood of acquiring melanoma. The good news is that the five-year survival rate is 99% if diagnosed and treated early.

- Non-Hispanic white folks have roughly a 30 times greater risk of skin cancer than non-Hispanic Black or Asian/Pacific Islander persons.
- Skin cancer in persons with a skin of color is generally identified at later stages when it's more difficult to treat. Some 25% of melanoma cases in African Americans are identified after the disease has spread to adjacent lymph nodes.

WHO IS MOST AT RISK FOR SKIN CANCER?

Although everyone may acquire skin cancer, you're at elevated risk if you:

- Spend a large amount of time working or playing in the sun.
- Get easily burnt; have a history of sunburns.
- Live in a sunny or high-altitude environment.
- Tan or utilize tanning beds.

- Have light-coloured eyes, blond or red hair and fair or freckled complexion.
- Have multiple moles or irregular-shaped moles.
- Have actinic keratosis (precancerous skin growths that are rough, scaly, dark pink-to-brown areas)
- Have a family history of skin cancer.
- Have had an organ transplant.
- Take drugs that inhibit or impair your immune system.
- Have been subjected to UV light treatment for treating skin disorders such as eczema or psoriasis.

WHERE DOES SKIN CANCER DEVELOP?

Skin cancer is most typically observed in sun-exposed parts of your skin – your face (including your lips), ears, neck, arms, chest, upper back, hands and legs. However, it may also form in less sun-exposed and more concealed regions of skin, including between your toes, beneath your fingernails, on the palms of your hands, soles of your feet and in your genital area.

WHERE, WITHIN THE SKIN LAYERS, DOES SKIN CANCER DEVELOP?

Where skin cancer arises — particularly, in which skin cells — is connected to the kinds and names of skin cancers.

Most skin malignancies develop in the epidermis, your skin's top layer. The epidermis has three primary cell types:

SQUAMOUS CELLS: These are flat cells in the outer section of the epidermis. They regularly shed as new cells arise. The skin cancer that may arise in these cells is termed squamous cell carcinoma.

BASAL CELLS: These cells lie underneath the squamous cells. They proliferate, reproduce and ultimately grow flatter and travel higher in the epidermis to create new squamous cells, replacing the dead squamous cells that have sloughed off. Skin cancer that develops in basal cells is termed basal cell carcinoma.

MELANOCYTES: These cells generate melanin, the brown pigment that gives skin its color and protects your skin from some of the sun's harmful UV rays. Skin cancer that develops in melanocytes is termed melanoma.

DOES SKIN CANCER AFFECT PEOPLE WITH SKIN OF COLOR?

People of all skin tones may acquire skin cancer. If you are a person of color, you may be less likely to have skin cancer because you have more of the brown pigment, melanin, in your skin.

Although less frequent than in nonwhite individuals, when skin cancer does form in people of color, it's generally diagnosed late and has a poorer prognosis. If you're Hispanic, the incidence of melanoma has climbed by 20% in the previous two decades. If you're Black and have melanoma, your five-year survival rate is 25% lower than it is for white individuals (67% versus 92%). Part of the explanation may be because it develops in less usual, less sun-exposed locations (it develops predominantly on palms of hands or soles of feet) and it's typically in late-stage when identified.

SYMPTOMS AND CAUSES
What Causes Skin Cancer?
The major cause of skin cancer is overexposure to sunlight, particularly when it results in sunburn and blistering. Ultraviolet (UV) rays from the sun break DNA in your skin, causing abnormal cells to grow. These aberrant cells quickly proliferate in a chaotic way, generating a mass of cancer cells.

Another cause of skin cancer is continuous skin contact with certain substances, such as tar and coal.

Many additional variables might raise your chance of acquiring skin cancer. See the question, "Who is most at risk for skin cancer?"

WHAT ARE THE SIGNS OF SKIN CANCER?

The most prevalent warning sign of skin cancer is a change on your skin, often a new growth, or a change in an existing growth or mole. The signs and symptoms of common and less frequent forms of skin malignancies are detailed here:

BASAL CELL CARCINOMA

Basal cell cancer is most typically observed on sun-exposed parts of the skin like your hands, face, arms, legs, ears, lips, and even bald places on the top of your head. Basal cell carcinoma is the most frequent kind of skin cancer in the globe. In most individuals, it's slow growing, typically doesn't spread to other regions of the body and is not life-threatening.

SIGNS AND SYMPTOMS OF BASAL CELL CARCINOMA INCLUDE:
- A little, smooth, pearly or waxy lump on the cheeks, ears, and neck.
- A flat, pink/red- or brown-coloured lesion on the trunk or arms and legs.
- Areas on the skin that appear like scars.
- Sores that seem crusty, have a depression in the centre or bleed regularly.

SQUAMOUS CELL CARCINOMA
Squamous cell carcinoma is most typically detected on sun-exposed parts of the skin like your hands, face, arms, legs, ears, lips, and even bald places on the top of your head. This skin cancer may also occur in

regions such as mucous membranes and genitals.

SIGNS AND SYMPTOMS OF SQUAMOUS CELL CARCINOMA INCLUDE:

- A hard pink or crimson nodule.
- A rough, scaly lesion that could itch, bleed and become crusty.

MELANOMA

Melanoma may develop in any place of your body. It may even build on your eyes and interior organs. The upper back is a popular location in males; the legs are a common spot in women. This is the most deadly sort of skin cancer since it may spread to other places in your body.

SIGNS AND SYMPTOMS OF MELANOMA INCLUDE:

- A brown-pigmented patch or bump.
- A mole that fluctuates in color, and size or that bleeds.

THINKING OF THE ABCDE RULE TELLS YOU WHAT SIGNS TO WATCH FOR:

- Asymmetry: uneven form.
- Border: fuzzy or unevenly formed margins.
- Color: mole with more than one color.
- Diameter: bigger than a pencil eraser (6 mm) .
- Evolution: growing, changing in form, color, or size. (This is the most essential indicator.)

Be attentive to pre-cancerous skin lesions that may develop into non-melanoma skin cancer. They appear as little scaly, tan or red patches, and are most typically seen on parts of the skin chronically exposed to the sun, such as the face and backs of the hands.

If you have a mole or other skin lesion that is giving you worry, schedule an appointment and present it to your healthcare professional. They will inspect your skin and may ask you to visit a dermatologist and have the lesion further analyzed.

WHAT ARE SOME OF THE LESSER-KNOWN SKIN CANCERS?
Some of the less frequent skin cancers include the following:

KAPOSI SARCOMA
Kaposi sarcoma is a rare malignancy most usually observed in patients who have impaired immune systems, those who have human immunodeficiency virus (HIV)/AIDS and those who are receiving immunosuppressant medicines and who have had an organ or bone marrow transplant.

SIGNS AND SYMPTOMS OF KAPOSI SARCOMA ARE:
- Blue, black, pink, red or purple flat or bumpy blotches or patches on your

arms, legs and face. Lesions could also form in your mouth, nose and throat.

MERKEL CELL CARCINOMA
Merkel cell carcinoma is a rare cancer that originates at the base of the epidermis, the top layer of your skin. This cancer develops in Merkel cells, which share the traits of nerve cells and hormone-making cells and are extremely near to the nerve ending in your skin. Merkel cell carcinoma is more prone to spread to other regions of the body than squamous or basal cell skin cancer.

SIGNS AND SYMPTOMS OF MERKEL CELL CARCINOMA ARE:
- A small reddish or purplish bump or lump on sun-exposed areas of skin.
- Lumps are fast-growing and can open up as ulcers or sores.

SEBACEOUS GLAND CARCINOMA
Sebaceous gland carcinoma is an uncommon, severe malignancy that

generally develops on your eyelid. This malignancy tends to form around your eyes since there's a big amount of sebaceous glands in that location.

SIGNS AND SYMPTOMS OF SEBACEOUS GLAND CARCINOMA ARE:
- A painless, round, firm, bump or lump on or slightly within your upper or lower eyelid.

DERMATOFIBROSARCOMA PROTUBERANS (DFSP)
DFSP is a rare skin cancer that originates in your dermis, the main layer of your skin. It develops slowly, seldom spreads and has a high survival rate.

SIGNS AND SYMPTOMS OF DFSP ARE:
- A purple, pink, red, or brown scar-like lump or rough elevated plaque on your skin.
- A birthmark-looking appearance in babies and youngsters.

DIAGNOSIS AND TESTS
How Is Skin Cancer Diagnosed?

First, your dermatologist may ask you whether you have observed any changes in any existing moles, freckles or other skin spots or if you've noticed any new skin growths. Next, your dermatologist will inspect all of your skin, including your scalp, ears, palms of your hands, soles of your feet, between your toes, around your genitals and between your buttocks.

If a skin lesion seems worrisome, a biopsy may be conducted. In a biopsy, a sample of tissue is extracted and transported to a laboratory to be studied under a microscope by a pathologist. Your dermatologist will inform you whether your skin lesion is skin cancer, and what kind you have and explain treatment choices.

MANAGEMENT AND TREATMENT
How Is Skin Cancer Treated?

Treatment varies with the stage of cancer. Stages of skin cancer vary from stage 0 to stage IV. The greater the number, the more cancer has spread.

Sometimes a biopsy alone may remove all the malignant tissue if the malignancy is tiny and localized to your skin's surface alone. Other frequent skin cancer therapies, performed alone or in combination, include:

CRYOTHERAPY
Cryotherapy employs liquid nitrogen to freeze skin cancer. The dead cells slough off the following therapy. Precancerous skin lesions termed actinic keratosis, and other tiny, early malignancies localized to the skin's top layer may be treated using this approach.

EXCISIONAL SURGERY
This procedure includes removing the tumor and some surrounding good skin to make sure all cancer has been eliminated.

MOHS SURGERY

With this treatment, the visible, elevated region of the tumor is removed first. Then your surgeon uses a knife to remove a small layer of skin cancer cells. The layer is studied under a microscope shortly after removal. Additional layers of tissue continue to be removed, one layer at a time until no more cancer cells are spotted under the microscope.

Mohs surgery eliminates only sick tissue, conserving as much surrounding normal tissue as possible. It's most typically used to treat basal cell and squamous cell malignancies and near sensitive or aesthetically significant regions, such as eyelids, ears, lips, forehead, scalp, fingers or genital area.

CURETTAGE AND ELECTRODESICCATION

The procedure employs a device with a sharp looping edge to remove cancer cells as it scrapes over the tumor. The region is then treated with an electric needle to remove any leftover cancer cells. This procedure is widely utilized for basal cell and squamous cell malignancies and precancerous skin lesions.

CHEMOTHERAPY AND IMMUNOTHERAPY

Chemotherapy employs drugs to destroy cancer cells. Anticancer treatments may be put directly on the skin (topical chemotherapy) if restricted to your skin's top layer or delivered by tablets or an IV if the cancer has spread to other regions of your body. Immunotherapy employs your own body's immune system to fight cancer cells.

RADIATION THERAPY

Radiation therapy is a method of cancer treatment that employs radiation (strong beams of energy) to destroy cancer cells or inhibit them from growing and dividing.

PHOTODYNAMIC THERAPY
In this treatment, your skin is covered with medicine and a blue or red fluorescent light then activates the drug. Photodynamic treatment eliminates precancerous cells while leaving normal cells alone.

PREVENTION
Can Skin Cancer Be Prevented?
In most situations, skin cancer may be avoided. The best approach to protect yourself is to avoid too much sunshine and sunburn. Ultraviolet (UV) rays from the sun harm your skin, and over time this may lead to skin cancer.

Ways to protect yourself against skin cancer include:
- Use a broad-spectrum sunscreen with a skin protection factor (SPF) of 30 or higher. Broad-spectrum sunscreens

protect against both UV-B and UV-A rays. Apply the sunscreen 30 minutes before you go outdoors. Wear sunscreen every day, especially on overcast days and throughout the winter months.

- Wear hats with broad brims to protect your face and ears.
- Wear long-sleeved shirts and slacks to protect your arms and legs. Look for garments with a UV protection factor marking for added protection.
- Wear sunglasses to protect your eyes. Look for glasses that block both UV-B and UV-A rays.
- Use a lip balm with sunscreen.
- Avoid the sun between 10 a.m. and 4 p.m.
- Avoid tanning beds. If you want a tanned appearance, apply a spray-on tanning product.
- Ask your healthcare practitioner or pharmacist whether any of the drugs you take make your skin more

susceptible to sunlight. Some medicines known to make your skin more susceptible to the sun include tetracycline and fluoroquinolone antibiotics, tricyclic antibiotics, the antifungal agent griseofulvin, and statin cholesterol-lowering pharmaceuticals.

- Check all the skin on your body and head for any changes in size, shape or color of skin growths or the formation of new skin spots. Don't forget to inspect your scalp, ears, the palms of your hands, soles of your feet, between your toes, your genital region and between your buttocks. Use mirrors and even snap images to assist in spotting changes in your skin over time. Make an appointment with your dermatologist if you observe any changes in a mole or other skin area.

OUTLOOK / PROGNOSIS

What Are The Prospects For Persons With Skin Cancer?

Nearly all skin cancers can be cured if they are treated before they have a chance to spread. The sooner skin cancer is identified and removed, the higher your chance for a complete recovery. Ninety per cent of patients with basal cell skin cancer are cured. It is crucial to continue following up with a dermatologist to make sure cancer does not recur. If anything appears incorrect, contact your doctor immediately away.

Most skin cancer fatalities are from melanoma. If you are diagnosed with melanoma:

- The five-year survival rate if it's discovered before cancer spreads to the lymph nodes is 99%.
- The five-year survival percentage, if it has migrated to neighbouring lymph nodes, is 66%.

- The five-year survival percentage, if it has progressed to distant lymph nodes and other organs, is 27%.

WHEN SHOULD I SEE MY HEALTHCARE PROVIDER?
Make an appointment to visit your healthcare practitioner or dermatologist as soon as you notice:

- Any changes to your skin or changes in the size, shape or color of existing moles or other skin problems.
- The look of new growth on your skin.
- A sore that doesn't heal.
- Spots on your skin that are distinct from others.
- Any patches that alter, itch or bleed.
- Your physician will evaluate your skin, take a biopsy (if required), make a diagnosis and discuss therapy. Also, consult your dermatologist yearly for a comprehensive skin evaluation.

WHAT QUESTIONS SHOULD I ASK MY HEALTHCARE PROVIDER?

Questions to ask your dermatologist may include:

- What form of skin cancer do I have?
- What stage is my skin cancer?
- What tests will I need?
- What's the best therapy for my skin cancer?
- What are the adverse effects of the treatment?
- What are the probable problems of this malignancy and the therapy for it?
- What result can I expect?
- Do I have an increased risk of further skin cancers?
- How frequently should I be seen for follow-up checkups?

FREQUENTLY ASKED QUESTIONS

How Can Skin Cancer Become A Life-threatening Malignancy?

You may ask how cancer on the surface of your skin becomes a life-threatening malignancy. It seems natural to imagine you could merely scrape off the skin containing the cancer cells or even remove the malignant skin lesion with a small skin surgery and that's all that would be required. These procedures are effectively employed if cancer is discovered early.

But if skin cancer isn't identified early, something that's "just on my skin" might develop and spread beyond the local region. Cancer cells break out and migrate through the bloodstream or lymph system. The cancer cells settle in other places in your body and proceed to proliferate and evolve into new tumors. This travel and spread is termed metastasis.

The kind of cancer cell where cancer initially originated — termed primary cancer — defines the type of cancer. For example, if malignant melanoma metastasized to the lungs, the cancer would still be labelled malignant melanoma. This is how that superficial skin cancer may grow into life-threatening malignancy.

WHY DOES SKIN CANCER OCCUR IN MORE NON-SUN-EXPOSED BODY AREAS IN PEOPLE OF COLOR?

Scientists don't entirely know why individuals with skin color acquire cancer in non-sun-exposed places, such as their hands and feet. They assume that the sun is less of an impact. However, doctors still encounter plenty of UV sunlight-induced melanomas and squamous cell skin cancer in persons of race, with skin tones ranging from fair to extremely dark.

ARE ALL MOLES CANCEROUS?

Most moles are not malignant. Some moles are present from birth, others develop up until roughly age 40. Most individuals have between 10 and 40 moles.

In rare situations, a mole may progress into melanoma. If you have more than 50 moles, you have an increased probability of acquiring melanoma.

CHAPTER 2

Debunking Common Myths/Misconceptions About Skin Cancer

It's crucial to protect your skin from the sun's damaging rays. That's because sun exposure may cause skin cancer, including melanoma—the most serious kind of skin cancer.

With melanoma, cancer cells develop on your skin, either in a new region or on or around an existing mole. When you identify these skin malignancies and get treatment promptly, they are generally curable. But untreated, they may spread to the lymph nodes and other organs and can lead to death.

MYTH: Skin cancer isn't hazardous
FACT: While certain forms of skin cancers are extremely curable and have great

survival rates, melanoma is the worst type of skin cancer. According to the American Cancer Society (ACS), melanoma diagnosis rates have climbed substantially over the previous several decades, and it forecasts that 7,650 people will die from it in 2022. Therefore, consulting a doctor for anything out of the norm is crucial.

MYTH: Melanoma is infrequent and primarily affects elderly individuals
FACT: The ACS anticipates that over 100,000 individuals will be diagnosed with this kind of skin cancer in 2022. They will join the more than 1 million individuals living with it. And although it's true that many of those folks are older, younger people aren't exempt. "It's one of the most frequent malignancies in young people, particularly young women,".

MYTH: People with darker skin don't acquire melanoma

FACT: "Melanoma does not discriminate,". People with pale skin and lighter eye color are actually at increased risk for this form of skin cancer. But it hits individuals of all ethnicities and skin hues. And persons with darker complexion are more commonly identified at a later stage of the illness (after it has spread) (after it has spread). Thus, they are less likely to withstand it than persons with lighter skin.

MYTH: Melanoma only attacks the skin
FACT: The skin is the most prevalent area for this form of cancer to grow. But it may also occur on the eyes, scalp, nails, feet and mucous membranes like the sinuses, inside of the nose or mouth, vagina and anus.

MYTH: Melanomas always look dark in color
FACT: Sometimes, these malignancies seem pink, red, purple or colorless. "A patch on your skin that is asymmetrical or has an

uneven border should still be looked out, no matter what color it is,".

MYTH: You'll only acquire melanoma if you've had years of sun exposure
FACT: This form of cancer is related to intermittent sun exposure throughout childhood and throughout your life. And just one blistering sunburn at a young age may boost the likelihood that you'll acquire skin cancer, while five or more blistering sunburns between ages 15 and 20 increases your risk by 80%.

MYTH: If you acquire melanoma, it's usually straightforward to treat
FACT: When you identify melanoma early, therapy may be quite uncomplicated. But when melanoma spreads to the liver, brain, bone or digestive system, it might need more invasive and long-term therapies, and it can be deadly.

MYTH: You don't need to apply sunscreen on overcast days

FACT: On overcast days, 80% of the sun's UV radiation may still reach your skin. Cloudy states like Washington, Oregon and Vermont have some of the highest incidences of melanoma. "Cloudy weather may offer individuals a false feeling of protection,".

MYTH: Your cosmetics offers adequate sun protection on your face

FACT: Most cosmetic products don't contain the necessary SPF of 30 or higher. And even if yours does, you're not receiving the protection you need unless you're reapplying it every two hours.

MYTH: You can achieve a safe tan using a tanning bed

FACT: According to the Skin Cancer Foundation, indoor tanning beds may release 10 to 15 times more UV radiation than the sun at its peak. Using a tanning bed before age 35 raises your chance of acquiring melanoma by 75%. And indoor tanning is connected to roughly 6,200 incidences of melanoma in the United States per year.

MYTH: A foundation tan may protect you from melanoma
FACT: When your skin changes color in reaction to sun exposure, that's an indication of damage. There is no such thing as a safe base tan. If you enjoy the look of tanned skin, pick a lotion or bronzer.

MYTH: You need sun exposure without sunscreen to receive the vitamin D you need
FACT: It's true that your skin will create vitamin D when you expose it to the sun without protection. But such exposure also raises your risk of skin cancer. "It's safer to acquire vitamin D from meals like milk and cereal items that have vitamin D added, or from supplements,".

MYTH: If you apply sunscreen, you're protected from skin cancer

FACT: Sunscreen is crucial, and you should apply a broad-spectrum sunscreen with an SPF of 30 or greater, reapplied every two hours, for UV protection. But sunscreen is simply one item that can help protect you. You should also avoid direct sunlight between 10 a.m. and 4 p.m., seek shade whenever you can, and wear a wide-brimmed hat and sunglasses that filter dangerous UV rays to minimize your skin cancer risk.

MYTH: Skin cancer only affects people with fair skin.

FACT: While people with fair skin are more susceptible to skin cancer, it can affect anyone regardless of skin tone.

MYTH: Skin cancer is not a serious condition.

FACT: Skin cancer, especially melanoma, can be deadly if not detected and treated early.

MYTH: Sunscreen is not necessary on cloudy days.
FACT: The sun's UV rays can still reach the earth on cloudy days, so it is important to use sunscreen even when it is cloudy.

MYTH: A base tan will protect you from getting burned.
FACT: A base tan does not provide adequate protection from the sun and can increase your risk of skin cancer.

MYTH: Skin cancer only occurs on areas of the skin that have been exposed to the sun.
FACT: Skin cancer can occur on any part of the body, including areas that are not typically exposed to the sun.

MYTH: Tanning beds are safe.

FACT: Tanning beds emit harmful UV rays that can increase the risk of skin cancer.

MYTH: Skin cancer is only a problem for older people.
FACT: While the risk of skin cancer increases with age, it can occur at any age. It is important for people of all ages to practice sun safety and protect their skin.

MYTH: Skin cancer only occurs in areas that are red or burned.
FACT: Skin cancer can occur on any part of the skin, regardless of whether it has been burned or not.

MYTH: If you have dark skin, you are not at risk for skin cancer.
FACT: While people with darker skin are less likely to develop skin cancer, it is still possible and it is important for everyone to practice sun safety.

MYTH: Skin cancer is rare.

FACT: Skin cancer is the most common type of cancer in the United States, with millions of cases diagnosed each year.

MYTH: You only need to wear sunscreen at the beach.
FACT: It is important to protect your skin from the sun's harmful UV rays whenever you are outside, even if you are not at the beach.

MYTH: You don't need to reapply sunscreen if you are not sweating or swimming.
FACT: Sunscreen should be reapplied every two hours, or immediately after swimming or sweating.

MYTH: Wearing clothes and a hat is enough protection from the sun.
FACT: While wearing protective clothing and a hat can help to reduce your risk of skin cancer, it is still important to use sunscreen to provide full protection.

MYTH: Skin cancer is not hereditary.
FACT: There is a genetic component to the risk of developing skin cancer, so people with a family history of skin cancer may be more likely to develop it themselves.

MYTH: Skin cancer is only caused by the sun.
FACT: While UV radiation from the sun is the main cause of skin cancer, it can also be caused by other sources of UV radiation such as tanning beds.

MYTH: If you have a lot of moles, you are at higher risk for skin cancer.
FACT: While having a lot of moles can increase the risk of skin cancer, it is more important to pay attention to the appearance and changes in individual moles rather than the total number.

MYTH: Skin cancer only affects the surface of the skin.

FACT: Skin cancer can spread to other parts of the body if it is not detected and treated early.

THE BOTTOM LINE

There are a lot of misconceptions about melanoma, and skin cancer in general. No one is immune to the disease, so it's crucial to examine your skin from head to toe every month. If you see a new mole, or a change in an existing mole, talk to a healthcare provider.

CHAPTER 3

Tips To Help Cope With Skin Cancer

SKIN CANCER EMOTIONAL WELL-BEING AND COPING STRATEGIES
- Dealing with the emotional effect of a skin cancer diagnosis
- Finding help from loved ones, support groups, or therapists
- Managing anxiety, stress, and sadness

Skin cancer may have a major emotional effect on persons who get a diagnosis. It may lead to emotions of worry, anxiety, despair, anger, and uncertainty about the future. Coping with the emotional components of skin cancer is vital for general well-being and may lead to improved treatment success. In this answer, we will examine the emotional well-being of persons with skin cancer and explore coping techniques for handling the accompanying issues.

DEALING WITH THE EMOTIONAL IMPACT OF A SKIN CANCER DIAGNOSIS: Receiving a skin cancer diagnosis may be distressing and may provoke a variety of emotional reactions. It is crucial to recognise and treat these feelings appropriately. Here are some strategies to consider:

ACKNOWLEDGE AND EXPRESS EMOTIONS: Allow yourself to feel and express your emotions. It is common to experience a variety of emotions, including fear, grief, anger, or irritation. Give yourself permission to experience these feelings and find appropriate methods to express them, such as talking to a trusted friend or family member, writing in a diary, or participating in creative activities like painting or music.

EDUCATE YOURSELF: Learning more about skin cancer, its therapies, and the prognosis may help ease worry and uncertainty.

Consult with your healthcare professional or seek credible sources of information to acquire a better knowledge of your situation. However, it is crucial to find a balance between being informed and avoiding excessive exposure to potentially disturbing material.

SEEK HELP: Reach out to your loved ones, friends, or support groups who may give emotional support during this tough time. Talking freely about your thoughts and worries with trustworthy folks may give comfort and help lessen stress.

Sharing your experiences with others who have gone through similar journeys in support groups may be very useful as they can give empathy, understanding, and practical assistance.

FINDING SUPPORT FROM LOVED ONES, SUPPORT GROUPS, OR THERAPISTS:

Support from numerous sources may substantially aid in emotional well-being when suffering from skin cancer. Consider the following options:

LOVED ONES: Lean on your family and close friends for emotional support. They may give a listening ear, provide support, accompany you to medical appointments, and aid you with practical problems. Sharing your thoughts and emotions with loved ones may improve your relationship and ease feelings of loneliness.

SUPPORT GROUPS: Joining a support group for those with skin cancer may be enormously useful. These groups give a safe area to share experiences, discuss coping skills, and obtain emotional support from people who can relate to your path. Local cancer clinics, hospitals, or internet communities may provide support group choices.

THERAPISTS OR COUNSELLORS: Professional assistance from therapists or counsellors who specialize in oncology or coping with chronic diseases may give significant support. They may help you process your emotions, create coping techniques, and give direction on managing stress and anxiety. Therapists may apply different methods such as cognitive-behavioral therapy (CBT) or mindfulness techniques to address particular emotional difficulties.

MANAGING ANXIETY, STRESS, AND DEPRESSION:
Skin cancer may lead to heightened worry, tension, and despair. Employing coping methods might help handle these feelings effectively:

COGNITIVE-BEHAVIORAL TECHNIQUES: Cognitive-behavioral therapy (CBT) may help patients recognize and fight negative thinking patterns related with their disease. This treatment focuses on reframing thinking, improving coping strategies, and boosting problem-solving abilities.

RELAXATION TECHNIQUES: Engaging in relaxation activities, such as deep breathing, progressive muscle relaxation, or guided imagery, may help decrease anxiety and generate a feeling of peace.

MINDFULNESS AND MEDITATION: Practicing mindfulness and meditation may promote emotional well-being by developing present-moment awareness, lowering stress, and enhancing general mental resilience.

PHYSICAL ACTIVITY: Regular exercise has been demonstrated to boost mood and decrease anxiety and sadness. Engaging in physical activities that fit your talents and interests may be a beneficial complement to your coping techniques.

SEEK PROFESSIONAL TREATMENT: If anxiety, stress, or depression become overpowering or interfere with your everyday life, consider obtaining professional help. A mental health expert may give treatment, administer appropriate drugs if required, and provide advice on coping techniques customized to your unique requirements.

KEEP EDUCATED BUT CREATE LIMITS: While it's necessary to keep informed about your health and therapy, it's also crucial to set boundaries for your emotional well-being. Limit exposure to disturbing content, avoid extensive online searches, and concentrate on dependable sources of information. This may help eliminate unneeded tension or dread.

Remember that everyone's experience with skin cancer is unique, and it's crucial to identify coping mechanisms that work best for you. Reach out for assistance when required, and take care of yourself holistically throughout your cancer experience.

SKIN CANCER SUN PROTECTION MEASURES
- **Importance of sun protection for avoiding further harm**
- **Tips for wearing sunscreen efficiently**
- **Wearing protective clothes and accessories**
- **Seeking cover during high sun hours**

It is crucial to use suitable sun protection measures to avoid additional damage to the skin and lower the chance of acquiring skin cancer. Here are some basic tips for protecting your skin from the damaging effects of the sun:

IMPORTANCE OF SUN PROTECTION:
Sun protection serves a critical function in avoiding additional damage to the skin. Prolonged and unprotected exposure to the

sun's UV rays may lead to many forms of skin cancer, including melanoma, basal cell carcinoma, and squamous cell carcinoma. By implementing sun protection measures, you may dramatically lower the likelihood of getting these illnesses. It is especially vital to protect the skin of youngsters since they are more vulnerable to sunburn and long-term harm.

TIPS FOR USING SUNSCREEN EFFECTIVELY:
Sunscreen is an essential component of any sun protection practice. Here are some recommendations for applying sunscreen effectively:

- Choose a broad-spectrum sunscreen that gives protection against both UVA and UVB radiation. Look for a sun protection factor (SPF) of 30 or greater.
- Apply sunscreen liberally to all exposed regions of the skin at least 15

to 30 minutes before going outdoors. Don't neglect typically ignored places like the ears, the back of the neck, and the tips of the feet.

- Reapply sunscreen every two hours, or more often if you are swimming or sweating hard.
- Pay attention to the expiry date of your sunscreen and replace it if it has expired.
- Remember that sunscreen is not a full barrier against the sun's damaging rays, thus it should be used in combination with other sun protection methods.
- Wearing Protective Clothing and Accessories:
- In addition to sunscreen, wearing protective clothes and accessories may considerably boost your sun protection. Here are some recommendations:
- Opt for clothes with a tight weave, such as long-sleeved shirts, long

trousers, and wide-brimmed caps. These devices create a physical barrier against the sun's rays and decrease direct exposure to the skin.

- Choose lightweight and breathable materials to remain cool and comfortable in hot weather.
- Look for clothes branded with an ultraviolet protection factor (UPF) rating, which shows the degree of UV protection it gives. Higher UPF ratings give more sun protection.
- Wear sunglasses that filter both UVA and UVB radiation to protect your eyes and the sensitive skin surrounding them.

SEEKING SHADE DURING PEAK SUN HOURS:
The sun's rays are brightest and most destructive between 10 a.m. and 4 p.m. During these peak hours, it is essential to seek shade as much as possible. This may help prevent direct exposure to UV radiation

and lower the risk of sunburn and skin damage.

When seeking shade, employ structures like umbrellas, canopies, or seek refuge behind trees or buildings. Even while in the shade, remember to continue utilizing additional sun protection measures like sunscreen and protective clothes, since UV radiation may still reach your skin indirectly.

In conclusion, protecting your skin from the sun is of essential significance to avoid additional damage and lower the chance of skin cancer. By following these sun protection practices, including the use of sunscreen, wearing protective clothes and accessories, and finding cover during peak sun hours, you may enjoy the outdoors safely and keep healthy skin. Remember to be proactive in protecting your skin and make sun protection a part of your everyday practice.

SKIN CANCER SKINCARE TIPS DURING AND AFTER TREATMENT
- Gentle skincare regimens for sensitive or impaired skin
- Choosing optimal skincare products and avoiding irritants
- Managing dryness, irritation, and other frequent adverse effects

Skin cancer is a dangerous disorder that needs early medical care. During and after skin cancer treatment, it is necessary to pay additional attention to skin care in order to promote healing, preserve the skin, and manage any side effects that may emerge. Here are some skincare advice for persons undergoing skin cancer treatment:

GENTLE SKINCARE PROCEDURES FOR DELICATE OR DAMAGED SKIN:
CLEANSE GENTLY: Use a gentle, fragrance-free cleanser that is particularly made for sensitive skin. Avoid strong soaps

or cleansers that may strip the skin of its natural oils.

BE AWARE OF WATER TEMPERATURE: Use lukewarm water while cleaning the skin to prevent additional dryness or irritation.

PAT DRY: After bathing, gently pat the skin dry with a soft towel. Avoid touching the skin, since this may create friction and increased discomfort.

MOISTURIZE REGULARLY: Apply a mild, fragrance-free moisturizer to the skin twice a day. Look for products that have calming ingredients like aloe vera or ceramides to help moisturize and restore the skin barrier. Choosing proper skincare products and avoiding irritants:

READ LABELS CAREFULLY: Look for products that are labelled as hypoallergenic, fragrance-free, and particularly developed for sensitive skin. Avoid items that include potentially irritating components such as alcohol, menthol, or strong perfumes.

PATCH TEST NEW PRODUCTS: Before applying a new product to your complete face or body, conduct a patch test on a small area of your skin to check for any unpleasant reactions or allergies.

SUN PROTECTION: It is vital to protect your skin from the sun's damaging UV rays, particularly during and after skin cancer treatment. Choose a broad-spectrum sunscreen with a high SPF and apply it liberally to all exposed regions of the skin. Additionally, wear protective clothing, a wide-brimmed hat, and seek shade whenever feasible.

MANAGING DRYNESS, ITCHING, AND OTHER FREQUENT SIDE EFFECTS:

HYDRATE FROM WITHIN: Drink lots of water to help keep your skin moisturized from the inside out.

USE MOISTURIZERS: Apply a moisturizer to wet skin after bathing or showering to seal in moisture.

AVOID HOT SHOWERS OR BATHS: Hot water may strip the skin of its natural oils, causing dryness and irritation. Opt for lukewarm water instead.

CALMING INGREDIENTS: Look for skincare products that have calming components such as oatmeal, chamomile, or calendula. These may help ease itching and reduce inflammation.

AVOID IRRITANTS: Avoid using abrasive exfoliants, toners, or astringents that might further irritate the skin. Stick to mild, fragrance-free products instead.

SEE YOUR HEALTHCARE PROVIDER: If you suffer severe or persistent side effects, such as excessive dryness, irritation, or skin reactions, see your healthcare provider for suitable treatment options.

Remember, everyone's skin is unique, so it's crucial to listen to your body and alter your skincare regimen appropriately. If you have any concerns or questions regarding skincare during or after skin cancer treatment, don't hesitate to contact your healthcare practitioner or dermatologist for tailored assistance.

BODY IMAGE AND SELF-ESTEEM
- Coping with changes in physical appearance
- Strategies for enhancing self-esteem and physical image
- Seeking professional assistance if required
Skin cancer may have a substantial influence on body image and self-esteem owing to the changes in physical appearance that may occur as a consequence of the

illness and its treatment. Coping with these changes may be tough, but there are ways that can help people raise their self-esteem and improve their body image. Seeking professional support, when required, is also a vital step in handling the emotional effect of skin cancer.

Skin cancer typically necessitates surgical procedures, which may result in scars, deformity, or the amputation of bodily parts, such as ears, nose, or limbs. Additionally, radiation treatment or chemotherapy might produce skin abnormalities including redness, peeling, or pigmentation problems. These physical abnormalities may be stressful and impair one's body image, resulting to a reduction in self-esteem and confidence.

coping with changes in physical appearance is a long process that involves both self-compassion and assistance from others. Here are some ways that may assist persons coping with skin cancer to increase their self-esteem and body image:

SELF-ACCEPTANCE AND SELF-COMPASSION: It is crucial to notice and accept the changes in physical appearance as a consequence of skin cancer. Practicing self-compassion means being compassionate and understanding toward oneself, rather than being too critical or judgemental.

EDUCATION AND KNOWLEDGE: Learning about the impacts of skin cancer therapy and the probable changes in physical appearance may help people better comprehend and come to terms with their condition. It may also relieve worries and misunderstandings, helping people to make educated choices regarding their self-care and treatment alternatives.

SEEKING SUPPORT: Connecting with individuals who have encountered similar issues may be useful. Support groups or online communities give a secure area to discuss experiences, feelings, and coping skills. Additionally, chatting with friends, relatives, or a therapist may give emotional support and help people process their emotions.

SELF-CARE AND GROOMING: Engaging in self-care activities that enhance physical and mental well-being may lead to a good body image. This might involve maintaining excellent hygiene, wearing comfortable clothing that makes one feel confident, and researching choices such as cosmetics, wigs, or prosthetics to improve the look if desired.

EMPHASIS ON STRENGTHS AND ACCOMPLISHMENTS: Shifting the emphasis from physical appearance to personal strengths, abilities, and achievements may assist increase self-esteem. Celebrating successes, making and attaining objectives, and participating in activities that offer pleasure and satisfaction may build a good self-image.

PRACTICING SELF-EXPRESSION: Engaging in activities that enable self-expression, such as painting, music, writing, or other creative outlets, may be therapeutic and help people reclaim a feeling of control and confidence in their identity.

HEALTHY LIFESTYLE: Taking care of one's physical health via regular exercise, a balanced diet, and adequate sleep may help with general well-being and a good body image. Physical exercise may also increase self-esteem by generating endorphins and fostering a feeling of achievement.

In certain circumstances, the emotional effect of skin cancer and changes in physical appearance may be overwhelming and need expert treatment. Mental health specialists, such as psychologists or therapists, may give advice, support, and specialized therapies to address body image problems, self-esteem difficulties, and any underlying anxiety or sadness. These specialists may help people develop coping mechanisms, manage emotions, and work towards creating a good self-image.

In conclusion, skin cancer may have a dramatic influence on body image and self-esteem because of the changes in physical appearance that may occur. Coping with these changes entails self-acceptance, finding support, practicing self-care, concentrating on strengths, and obtaining professional assistance when required. By taking efforts to address body image problems and promote self-esteem, people may improve their general well-being and adapt to the difficulties of living with skin cancer.

FINDING SUPPORT IN YOUR COMMUNITY

- Connecting with local organizations or cancer support groups
- Engaging in activities and events that promote awareness and education
- Sharing experiences and learning from those who have had similar problems

Finding support for skin cancer in your community is vital for both sufferers and their loved ones. Dealing with a cancer diagnosis may be difficult, but connecting with local groups, partaking in awareness activities, and sharing stories can give essential support and resources. Here's a full summary of these three approaches:

CONNECTING WITH LOCAL ORGANIZATIONS OR CANCER SUPPORT GROUPS:
a. RESEARCH: Start by exploring local organizations or cancer support groups that primarily concentrate on skin cancer. Look for trustworthy groups like the American

Cancer Society (ACS) or the Skin Cancer Foundation, which typically have local branches or affiliations.

b. ONLINE RESOURCES: Visit their websites or contact them to learn about the services they provide. Many organizations offer resources such as instructional materials, helplines, internet forums, and support group listings.

c. SUPPORT GROUP MEETINGS: Attend support group meetings arranged by local groups. These gatherings provide a secure and inviting atmosphere where persons impacted by skin cancer may interact with others who understand their problems. Support group participants typically share stories, discuss coping tactics, and give emotional support.

d. ONLINE COMMUNITIES: Explore online communities and forums devoted to skin cancer. Websites like the Cancer Support

Community (CSC) or Inspire give venues where people may connect, share their experiences, ask questions, and get support from others in similar circumstances.

ENGAGING IN ACTIVITIES AND EVENTS THAT PROMOTE AWARENESS AND EDUCATION:

a. SKIN CANCER SCREENINGS: Stay informed about local activities that provide free or cheap skin cancer screenings. These screenings can identify possible skin cancer at an early stage and give a chance to learn more about preventative and self-examination practices.

b. AWARENESS PROGRAMS: Participate in local skin cancer awareness programs. These campaigns may involve activities such as walks, runs, or fundraising events aimed at raising awareness and funding for skin cancer research and support services.

c. EDUCATIONAL WORKSHOPS AND SEMINARS: Attend workshops and seminars offered by local healthcare institutions, dermatological clinics, or cancer support groups. These programs generally address subjects including skin cancer prevention, screening, treatment choices, and coping techniques. They give a chance to learn from medical experts and meet with individuals in the community who are interested in skin cancer activism.

SHARING EXPERIENCES AND LEARNING FROM OTHERS:

a. SUPPORT GROUP TALKS: Engage in open and honest talks during support group gatherings. By sharing your experiences and problems, you might obtain insights from others who have had similar circumstances. Listening to others' tales may also bring consolation, support, and alternate viewpoints.

b. ONLINE SUPPORT FORUMS: Participate in online support forums and discuss your story with skin cancer. By sharing your experiences, you may contribute to a helpful online community and perhaps assist others going through similar issues.

c. PEER MENTORING: Seek for chances for peer mentoring programs within your local community or via national organizations. These programs link persons who have just been diagnosed with skin cancer with survivors who can give advice, support, and personal experience of navigating the process.

d. COUNSELING SERVICES: Consider obtaining professional counseling services, such as therapy or counseling sessions given by healthcare institutions or cancer support groups. These programs may give a safe area to vent feelings, address issues, and learn coping methods from experienced specialists.

Remember, seeking support for skin cancer in your community is a continuous journey. Stay connected with local organizations, attend events, and actively participate in support groups to ensure you have a network of resources and a supportive community to depend on during your journey.

PLANNING FOR THE FUTURE
- Understanding the need for frequent check-ups and screenings
- Managing long-term care and survival
- Taking efforts to limit the chance of skin cancer recurrence

Planning for the future is vital when it comes to controlling and preventing skin cancer. By executing a thorough strategy, people may boost their odds of early diagnosis, successfully manage long-term care, and lower the risk of cancer recurrence. Here's a full review of the essential elements to consider while preparing for the future of skin cancer:

UNDERSTANDING THE IMPORTANCE OF REGULAR CHECK-UPS AND SCREENINGS:
Regular check-ups and screenings are crucial for discovering skin cancer at its earlier stages when it is most curable. Dermatologists urge that people undertake frequent self-examinations of their skin and undergo a professional skin examination at least once a year. During these check-ups, dermatologists might spot problematic moles or abnormalities that may need additional study. By knowing the value of frequent tests, people may remain cautious and discover any possible skin cancer early.

MANAGING LONG-TERM CARE AND SURVIVORSHIP:

For patients who have been diagnosed with skin cancer, adequate long-term care and survivorship management are vital. This involves following up with the healthcare team, attending frequent follow-up visits, and sticking to approved treatment programs.

Dermatologists and oncologists will evaluate the individual's progress, check for recurrence, and manage any possible side effects or consequences from therapy. Developing a strong support network, including healthcare professionals, family, and friends, may also give emotional and practical help throughout the survival journey.

TAKING STEPS TO REDUCE THE RISK OF SKIN CANCER RECURRENCE:

After completing treatment for skin cancer, it is crucial to take preventive steps to limit the chance of recurrence. Here are some strategies to consider:

a. SUN PROTECTION: Practicing sun protection is crucial in avoiding additional harm to the skin. This involves wearing protective clothes, applying a broad-spectrum sunscreen with a high SPF, finding cover during peak sun hours, and wearing sunglasses and hats.

b. AVOIDING TANNING BEDS: Tanning beds produce dangerous ultraviolet (UV) radiation, which raises the risk of skin cancer. It is vital to avoid using tanning beds and opt for safer options, such as self-tanning products.

c. REGULAR SKIN CHECKS: Continuing to do self-examinations and monitoring the skin for any changes is vital, even after therapy. Promptly reporting any worrisome moles or lesions to the dermatologist might assist in early diagnosis and treatment if required.

d. HEALTHY LIFESTYLE: Maintaining a healthy lifestyle may help general well-being and lessen the chance of skin cancer recurrence. This involves adopting a balanced diet, participating in regular exercise, regulating stress levels, and avoiding tobacco and excessive alcohol usage.

In addition to the aforementioned, remaining updated about the newest research and breakthroughs in skin cancer treatment and prevention is vital. Medical advances, new treatment choices, and upcoming technology may profoundly affect future planning and decision-making. It is recommended to speak with healthcare specialists that specialize in skin cancer to build a customised approach that meets individual requirements and circumstances.

Remember, skin cancer is a very preventable and curable disorder when caught early. By actively preparing for the future and executing preventative actions, people may dramatically lessen the burden of skin cancer on their lives and improve their long-term prognosis.

SEX & RELATIONSHIP

Handling sexual concerns in skin cancer patients involves empathy, understanding, and a multidisciplinary approach incorporating the patient's healthcare team. Skin cancer and its therapies may have physical, emotional, and psychological consequences on people, which may influence their sexual health and relationships. Here are some recommendations to assist address and manage sexual difficulties in skin cancer patients:

OPEN COMMUNICATION: Encourage patients to freely communicate their worries and sexual difficulties with their healthcare staff. Creating a comfortable and non-judgmental atmosphere helps patients to communicate their problems, fears, and questions relating to sexual health.

EDUCATE PATIENTS: Provide patients with appropriate information regarding the possible effect of skin cancer and its therapies on sexual health. Explain the possible physical and psychological changes they may encounter, such as changes in body image, scars, exhaustion, or discomfort.

ADDRESS BODY IMAGE CONCERNS: Skin cancer and its treatments may lead to apparent changes in appearance, including scarring, deformity, or hair loss. Such changes may impair body image and self-esteem, hurting sexual confidence and intimacy. Encourage patients to voice their thoughts and give them tools to assist manage body image problems, such as support groups or counseling services.

ENCOURAGE SELF-CARE AND SELF-ACCEPTANCE: Promote self-care behaviors that may enhance body image and self-confidence. Encourage patients to participate in things they love, such as exercise, hobbies, or pampering themselves. Emphasize the value of self-acceptance and self-love, reminding patients that their worth is not primarily determined by their physical appearance.

MANAGE TREATMENT SIDE EFFECTS: Some skin cancer therapies, such as surgery, radiation therapy, or chemotherapy, might have physical side effects that may influence sexual function and desire. Collaborate with the healthcare team to handle these side effects properly. For example, if a woman develops vaginal dryness owing to hormonal changes, a gynecologist may prescribe topical moisturizers or propose hormonal therapy.

PROVIDE SEXUAL HEALTH RESOURCES: Refer patients to sexual health professionals or counselors who are skilled in dealing with cancer patients. These specialists may give specialized help, therapy, and solutions to handle sexual disorders efficiently. They may also give information on sexual aids, strategies, and exercises to increase intimacy.

EXPLORE ALTERNATE KINDS OF INTIMACY: In circumstances when sexual activity may not be feasible or pleasant, urge patients to explore alternative types of intimacy and connection with their partners. This might entail emotional connection, non-sexual physical intimacy, or developing new methods of pleasuring each other.

SUPPORT PSYCHOLOGICAL WELL-BEING: Emotional support is vital in handling sexual difficulties. Encourage patients to seek therapy or support groups to address any emotional or psychological issues they may be encountering. Mental health practitioners may give coping skills, stress management techniques, and advice on strengthening intimacy within the setting of cancer treatment.

INCLUDE PARTNERS: Encourage patients to include their partners in conversations about sexual health. Partners may give emotional support and assist to discovering answers together. Open communication and collaborative decision-making may develop a deeper link between couples during this hard period.

LONG-TERM FOLLOW-UP: Sexual difficulties may remain or alter over time, even after the end of skin cancer therapy. Therefore, it is necessary to schedule frequent follow-up sessions to check and manage any persisting difficulties linked to sexual health.

Remember, each individual's experience with skin cancer and its influence on sexual health is unique. Tailor your approach to fit the individual requirements and concerns of each patient. Collaborating with a multidisciplinary healthcare team, including oncologists, dermatologists, psychologists, and sexual health professionals, is crucial in delivering complete treatment for skin cancer patients struggling with sexual disorders.

QUESTIONS SKIN CANCER PATIENTS CAN ASK THEIR HEALTH PROVIDER:

- What is the stage of my skin cancer?
- What form of skin cancer do I have?
- What treatment options are available for my particular form of skin cancer?
- How effective are these therapy options?
- What adverse effects might I anticipate from treatment?

- How will therapy affect my everyday life and routine?
- Can I work throughout treatment?
- Will I need to have surgery?
- How long will therapy last?
- Will I need follow-up care or monitoring following treatment?
- Can my skin cancer be cured?
- What is the prognosis for my particular form of skin cancer?
- Are there any clinical trials or experimental therapies I may engage in?
- How can I effectively treat my skin cancer at home?
- Is there any lifestyle or food adjustments I may make to enhance my outcome?
- How can I avoid future skin cancers?
- What should I do if I see any changes or new spots on my skin?
- How frequently should I receive skin cancer screenings?

- How can I lower my chance of having skin cancer?
- What is the importance of sun protection in skin cancer prevention?
- What is the function of genetics in skin cancer development?
- How can I spot the early indications of skin cancer?
- Can skin cancer travel to other regions of my body?
- Will I need to undergo chemotherapy or radiation therapy?
- How will therapy change my appearance?
- How will therapy affect my quality of life?
- How can I control pain or discomfort during the treatment?
- How can I gain assistance from friends and family throughout treatment?
- Are there any financing options or support available to help me manage treatment costs?

- Can I continue to work or engage in typical activities throughout treatment?
- How will therapy affect my physical and mental well-being?
- Are there any support groups or counselling services accessible to me throughout treatment?
- Can I continue to take my normal meds while having treatment?
- What should I do if I suffer any unpleasant side effects from treatment?
- How can I contact my healthcare team about my concerns or questions?
- What are the long-term implications of therapy on my skin cancer?
- How can I treat my skin cancer in the future to avoid recurrence?
- Can I anticipate having any physical limits following treatment?
- How can I keep updated about the latest research and breakthroughs in skin cancer treatment?

- Is there anything more I should know or ask about my skin cancer treatment and care?

CHAPTER 4

Complementary & Alternative Treatments For Skin Cancer

INTRODUCTION TO COMPLEMENTARY AND ALTERNATIVE TREATMENTS FOR SKIN CANCER

Skin cancer is a widespread kind of cancer that originates when abnormal cells in the skin proliferate uncontrolled. It is generally caused by exposure to ultraviolet (UV) light from the sun or artificial sources, such as tanning beds.

Traditional therapies for skin cancer include surgery, radiation therapy, chemotherapy, and targeted therapy. However, some people seek complementary and alternative therapies (CAM) alongside or instead of traditional techniques.

Complementary and alternative therapies relate to a varied variety of medical and healthcare techniques that are not normally considered part of traditional medicine. These therapies attempt to offer supportive care, boost well-being, and improve the overall quality of life. It is crucial to highlight that although certain CAM therapies may give advantages for symptom management, they are not alternatives for evidence-based medical treatments.

HERE ARE SOME TYPICAL COMPLEMENTARY AND ALTERNATIVE THERAPIES THAT PERSONS WITH SKIN CANCER MAY CONSIDER:

HERBAL AND NUTRITIONAL SUPPLEMENTS: Certain herbs and supplements are claimed to contain anti-cancer qualities. Examples include green tea, turmeric, vitamin D, selenium, and others. However, it is vital to talk with a healthcare practitioner before introducing any supplements into your regimen, since they may interfere with conventional therapies or have bad effects.

ACUPUNCTURE: Acupuncture is an ancient Chinese treatment that includes the insertion of tiny needles into particular spots on the body. It is said to enhance energy flow and facilitate healing. While acupuncture may not directly cure skin cancer, it may help control treatment-related symptoms such as pain, nausea, and exhaustion.

MIND-BODY METHODS: Various mind-body activities, such as meditation, yoga, and relaxation methods, may help decrease stress, anxiety, and enhance general well-being. These practices may be useful for those undergoing skin cancer therapy since they improve relaxation and mental clarity.

MASSAGE THERAPY: Massage therapy includes the manipulation of soft tissues to enhance circulation, relieve muscular tension, and induce relaxation. It may be effective for controlling treatment side effects, lowering anxiety, and boosting overall comfort.

HOMEOPATHY: Homeopathy is founded on the premise of "like cures like," utilizing very diluted chemicals to promote the body's natural healing reaction. However, the effectiveness of homeopathy in treating cancer remains debatable, and it should not be utilized as a primary therapy for skin cancer.

TRADITIONAL CHINESE MEDICATION (TCM): TCM comprises a variety of treatments, including herbal medication, acupuncture, nutritional therapy, and qi gong exercises. It offers a holistic approach to treatment, concentrating on restoring balance and fostering general well-being. TCM may be used as a supplemental therapy with conventional therapies.

It is crucial for persons contemplating complementary and alternative therapy for skin cancer to discuss it freely with their healthcare team. It is not suggested to entirely depend on CAM treatments for cancer therapy, since they lack strong scientific proof and may delay or interfere with appropriate medical measures. Integrating CAM methods should be done under the direction and supervision of a skilled healthcare provider who is educated about both conventional and alternative therapy.

In conclusion, complementary and alternative therapies may play a supporting role in controlling symptoms, enhancing well-being, and improving the quality of life for patients with skin cancer. However, they should be used in combination with evidence-based medical therapies and under the advice of healthcare specialists. It is vital to emphasize the safety and efficacy of therapies to guarantee the best potential results for skin cancer patients.

COMPLEMENTARY THERAPIES FOR SKIN CANCER: AN OVERVIEW

HERBAL REMEDIES AND BOTANICALS FOR SKIN CANCER TREATMENT

Complementary therapies relate to a varied variety of treatments and practices that are utilized alongside traditional medical treatments to promote and improve general well-being.

When it comes to skin cancer, complementary treatments may play a supporting role in treating symptoms, increasing the quality of life, and promoting the body's natural healing processes.

One type of alternative treatment that has attracted interest is herbal medicines and botanicals. While it's crucial to remember that these therapies should never replace established medical treatments for skin cancer, they may give extra advantages when used in combination with traditional procedures.

Herbal treatments and botanicals have been utilized for ages in numerous civilizations for their medical benefits. Some of these compounds have shown promise in laboratory investigations and early clinical trials for their potential anti-cancer properties. However, it's vital to approach these treatments with care, since the scientific data supporting their effectiveness and safety in treating skin cancer is currently limited. It's crucial to check with a healthcare practitioner before adopting any alternative therapy into your treatment plan.

HERE ARE A FEW HERBAL TREATMENTS AND BOTANICALS THAT HAVE BEEN EXAMINED FOR THEIR POSSIBLE IMPACT ON SKIN CANCER:

GREEN TEA: Green tea includes substances called polyphenols, notably catechins, which exhibit antioxidant and anti-inflammatory effects. Some studies show that these chemicals may help inhibit the development and spread of skin cancer cells. However, further study is required to discover the best dose, safety, and efficacy of green tea as a supplemental treatment for skin cancer.

CURCUMIN: Curcumin is the active element found in turmeric, a spice often used in Indian cuisine. Curcumin has exhibited anti-cancer capabilities in laboratory experiments, including the capacity to suppress the development of skin cancer cells. However, its poor bioavailability and restricted absorption in the body pose problems for its therapeutic usage. Researchers are studying alternative formulations and delivery ways to boost curcumin's efficiency as a possible therapy option.

ALOE VERA: Aloe vera gel is well renowned for its soothing and therapeutic capabilities, especially for skin-related problems. Some research shows that aloe vera may have anti-cancer actions and might help limit the proliferation of skin cancer cells. It may also give relief from radiation-induced skin damage and irritation. However, more clinical studies are essential to confirm its effectiveness and safety as a supplementary treatment for skin cancer.

BLACK RASPBERRY: Black raspberries are high in anthocyanins, a group of antioxidants that have shown promise in preventing and treating several forms of cancer. Some research have explored the effects of black raspberry extracts on skin cancer, revealing a decrease in tumor development and the activation of apoptosis (programmed cell death) in cancer cells. However, further study is required to verify these results and discover the best dose and composition.

MILK THISTLE: Milk thistle (Silybum marianum) includes a flavonoid compound known as silymarin, which has antioxidant and anti-inflammatory activities. While its major usage is treating liver disorders, several studies have shown that milk thistle may have potential anti-cancer properties. Research on its particular involvement in skin cancer therapy is limited, and additional research is necessary to determine its safety and effectiveness.

It's crucial to understand that herbal treatments and botanicals are not controlled in the same manner as pharmaceutical pharmaceuticals. The concentration and purity of active substances might vary greatly amongst products, making it vital to find reliable sources and check with a healthcare practitioner before usage. Additionally, herbal medicines might conflict with some prescriptions, so it's crucial to declare their usage to your healthcare professional.

In conclusion, herbal remedies and botanicals have shown promise in laboratory studies as potential complementary therapies for skin cancer. However, more rigorous research, including large-scale clinical trials, is necessary to validate their efficacy, safety, and optimal usage. It's crucial to approach these therapies with caution and contact your healthcare provider where necessary.

PHOTODYNAMIC THERAPY AS AN ALTERNATIVE SKIN CANCER TREATMENT

Photodynamic therapy (PDT) is an innovative and successful alternative treatment for some forms of skin cancer. It includes the use of a photosensitizing chemical, a particular kind of light, and oxygen to selectively target malignant cells while minimizing harm to healthy tissue. PDT has gained popularity owing to its non-invasive nature, few side effects, and excellent success rates in treating skin cancer.

The method of photodynamic treatment starts with the introduction of a photosensitizing agent. This agent is often a light-sensitive medicine that is either given topically to the skin or injected intravenously, depending on the kind and location of the skin cancer being treated. The photosensitizing substance is absorbed by the malignant cells over a particular length of time, whereas normal cells absorb a considerably lower quantity or none at all.

After an adequate incubation time, the targeted region is exposed to a precise wavelength of light that matches the absorption spectra of the photosensitizing chemical. This light may be obtained from many sources, such as lasers or light-emitting diodes (LEDs), and is often focused directly on the tumor or region of concern. The light activates the photosensitizing agent, causing a sequence of events that create reactive oxygen species (ROS), such as singlet oxygen, which are harmful to the cancer cells.

The ROS created during PDT inflicts harm on the malignant cells in numerous ways. Firstly, they generate oxidative stress, resulting in the breakdown of cellular components required for life. Secondly, the ROS may directly damage the blood arteries supporting the tumor, so reducing its nutritional and oxygen supply. Finally, the immune system is triggered by the production of damage-associated molecular patterns (DAMPs), resulting in an immunological response that assists in the killing of the cancer cells.

One of the primary benefits of photodynamic treatment is its selectivity for cancer cells. Normal cells that have not absorbed the photosensitizing chemical are little impacted by the light activation, lowering the chance of undesirable consequences and injury to healthy tissue. This selectivity makes PDT especially effective for treating superficial skin malignancies, such as basal cell carcinoma and squamous cell carcinoma.

PDT provides various advantages as an alternative skin cancer therapy. Firstly, it is a very non-invasive operation, often conducted on an outpatient basis, which means it does not need surgery. This makes it an intriguing choice for people who are not good candidates for surgery or want a less intrusive method. Additionally, PDT has a faster recovery period compared to surgical procedures, enabling patients to resume their daily activities more quickly.

Another benefit of PDT is its aesthetic result. Since the process specifically targets cancer cells without considerable harm to healthy tissue, it frequently results in great aesthetic outcomes with minimum scarring.

This is particularly crucial for treating skin malignancies situated in aesthetically sensitive locations, such as the face.

While PDT is typically well-tolerated, it may induce transitory adverse effects such as redness, edema, and discomfort at the treatment site. These effects are often modest and fade within a few days or weeks. The photosensitivity generated by the photosensitizing agent may necessitate patients to avoid direct sunlight or strong interior lights for a set time after treatment to prevent skin responses.

In conclusion, photodynamic therapy is an effective and promising alternative treatment for some forms of skin cancer. Its ability to specifically target cancer cells, minimum invasiveness, excellent aesthetic results, and low risk of side effects make it an appealing alternative for patients seeking non-surgical therapy. However, it is necessary to contact a healthcare practitioner to evaluate whether PDT is a good treatment choice depending on the precise kind, size, and location of the skin cancer.

ACUPUNCTURE AND TRADITIONAL CHINESE MEDICINE IN SKIN CANCER CARE

Acupuncture and Traditional Chinese Medicine (TCM) may have a complementary role in the treatment and management of skin cancer. While they are not alternatives to traditional medical treatments, they may be used as adjunct therapies to boost general well-being, relieve side effects, and enhance the body's natural healing processes.

Acupuncture is a crucial component of TCM, which has been practiced for thousands of years in China and other areas of East Asia. It includes the insertion of thin, sterile needles into precise spots on the body to promote and balance the flow of energy, or qi. According to TCM principles, when the body's qi is obstructed or unbalanced, it may lead to different health diseases, including skin illnesses such as skin cancer.

When it comes to skin cancer treatment, acupuncture may give various advantages. Firstly, it is known to induce relaxation and decrease tension, which may be especially useful for people undergoing cancer treatment. Stress reduction may assist improve general well-being and strengthen the body's capacity to deal with the problems connected with skin cancer.

Additionally, acupuncture has been observed to have analgesic, or pain-relieving, benefits. Skin cancer therapies, such as surgery, radiation therapy, or chemotherapy, may sometimes cause discomfort or suffering. Acupuncture may help ease these symptoms, lowering the dependency on pain drugs and enhancing the patient's quality of life.

Furthermore, acupuncture is supposed to boost the body's immunological system. It may increase immune activity and encourage a better response to skin cancer therapy. This may lead to better results and speedier recovery.

In TCM, the skin is considered a representation of the internal organs and general health. TCM practitioners frequently adopt a holistic approach, concentrating on the underlying imbalances that may contribute to the development or spread of skin cancer. They may analyze the patient's general health, lifestyle, and constitution to establish a specific treatment strategy.

Herbal medicine is another major part of TCM. Herbal medicines may be given to address particular imbalances, promote the body's natural healing processes, and lessen adverse effects associated with skin cancer therapy. Certain herbs have shown promise in reducing the development of cancer cells or enhancing the body's capacity to fight cancer.

It is crucial to emphasize that although acupuncture and TCM may offer supportive care for skin cancer patients, they are not alternatives for traditional medical therapies like surgery, radiation therapy, or chemotherapy. It is vital for patients to speak with their oncologists and dermatologists to ensure that they get the most suitable and successful therapies for their disease.

When seeking acupuncture or TCM for skin cancer treatment, it is recommended to choose a skilled and licensed practitioner with expertise in oncology support. They may work in concert with the patient's medical team to design a thorough treatment plan that meets the particular requirements and objectives of the client.

In summary, acupuncture and TCM may serve as helpful adjuvant therapy in skin cancer management. They may give advantages such as stress reduction, pain alleviation, immune system support, and general well-being. However, it is crucial to combine these therapies with traditional medical treatments to guarantee complete and successful care for skin cancer patients.

HOMEOPATHIC REMEDIES FOR SKIN CANCER: EFFICACY AND SAFETY CONSIDERATIONS

Skin cancer is a dangerous medical disorder defined by the uncontrolled proliferation of abnormal skin cells. It is often caused by excessive exposure to ultraviolet (UV) light from the sun or tanning beds. While standard medical therapies including surgery, radiation therapy, and chemotherapy are widely used to treat skin cancer, some patients may explore alternative techniques such as homeopathy.

Homeopathy is a comprehensive approach to medicine that strives to activate the body's intrinsic healing power. Homeopathic medicines are drawn from natural components and are manufactured in a very diluted form. The core concept of homeopathy is "like cures," which implies that a drug that generates symptoms in a healthy person may be administered in a very diluted form to treat comparable symptoms in a sick person.

When it comes to skin cancer, it is vital to highlight that homeopathy should not be utilized as a single or main therapeutic choice. Skin cancer is a potentially life-threatening disorder that needs prompt medical treatment and correct management by a competent healthcare practitioner. Homeopathic medicines may be used as an adjunctive or supportive therapy with conventional therapies, but they should not replace regular medical care.

That being said, certain homeopathic treatments may be utilized to ease some symptoms connected with skin cancer or to enhance general well-being. It is necessary to visit with a trained homeopathic practitioner who can personalize the therapy to your unique requirements. Here are a few homeopathic treatments that are occasionally used in skin cancer management:

THUJA OCCIDENTALIS: This medicine is produced from the Thuja tree and is often used in homeopathy for many skin diseases, including warts and some forms of skin malignancies. It is considered to have anti-viral and immune-stimulating effects.

CARCINOSIN: Carcinosin is a treatment obtained from malignant cells. It is widely used in homeopathy to maintain general vitality and balance in patients with a history of cancer or a propensity to cancer.

ARSENICUM ALBUM: Arsenicum album is a mineral-based medicine that is occasionally used in homeopathy for its anti-inflammatory and anti-itching effects. It may be beneficial in controlling cutaneous symptoms linked with cancer, such as itching, burning, and inflammation.

CALENDULA OFFICINALIS: Calendula, or marigold, is a plant-based treatment that is recognized for its wound-healing abilities. It may be administered topically as a cream or ointment to promote the healing of surgical wounds or skin ulcers associated with skin cancer therapy.

GRAPHITES: Graphites is a mineral-based treatment that may be effective for dry, scaly skin disorders typically observed in some kinds of skin cancer.

It is vital to note that there is minimal scientific data supporting the usefulness of homeopathic treatments in treating skin cancer. Homeopathy is typically regarded as a contentious issue in the medical world owing to the absence of rigorous scientific research confirming its usefulness. Therefore, it is vital to prioritize evidence-based conventional therapies and confer with a healthcare expert before contemplating any complementary or alternative techniques.

Furthermore, safety is a key worry when it comes to homeopathic therapies for skin cancer. Homeopathic treatments are often very diluted and generally regarded as safe when administered carefully. However, it is crucial to verify that the cures are bought from credible sources and that they are free from contaminants. Additionally, if you are having conventional treatments for skin cancer, it is vital to notify your healthcare practitioner about any homeopathic medicines you are using to prevent any interactions or harmful effects.

In summary, homeopathic treatments are not backed by scientific data for the treatment of skin cancer. The conventional treatment choices supplied by medical specialists have been carefully examined and confirmed effective. Relying on homeopathy alone for skin cancer therapy may be damaging to one's health and raise the chance of disease development. It is crucial to prioritize evidence-based medical procedures and consult with a healthcare expert for proper diagnosis and treatment.

AYURVEDIC PRACTICES AND SKIN CANCER MANAGEMENT

Ayurveda is an ancient Indian system of medicine that focuses on maintaining a balance between the body, mind, and spirit to promote general health and well-being. In Ayurveda, the focus is on preventive and holistic methods of treatment, including the care of numerous ailments, including skin cancer. While Ayurveda may not be the main treatment for skin cancer, it may be utilized as a complementary therapy to augment contemporary medical therapies and increase general well-being.

Ayurvedic treatments for skin cancer care concentrate upon the concepts of cleansing, immune system support, and preserving the balance of the doshas (vata, pitta, and kapha). Here are some typical Ayurvedic techniques and treatments used in the management of skin cancer:

HERBAL REMEDIES: Ayurveda incorporates a broad variety of herbs with possible anti-cancer qualities. Some widely used herbs for skin cancer therapy include turmeric (Curcuma longa), neem (Azadirachta indica), ashwagandha (Withania somnifera), guduchi (Tinospora cordifolia), and aloe vera (Aloe barbadensis). These plants are considered to offer antioxidant, anti-inflammatory, and immune-modulatory effects.

DETOXIFICATION: Ayurveda stresses the removal of toxins from the body as a strategy to promote healing and general health. Panchakarma, a detoxifying therapy, is widely advised in Ayurvedic skin cancer management. It incorporates numerous treatments like herbal massages, steam therapy (swedana), medicated enemas (basti), and nasal administration of herbal oils (nasya) to expel toxins and restore equilibrium.

DIETARY CHANGES: Ayurvedic practitioners may propose dietary alterations to help the treatment of skin cancer. This often means ingesting fresh and organic fruits and vegetables, whole grains, healthy fats, and lean meats. Foods high in antioxidants, such as berries, leafy greens, and turmeric, may be promoted owing to their possible anti-cancer qualities.

LIFESTYLE MODIFICATIONS: Ayurveda lays significant focus on keeping a healthy lifestyle. This involves adopting stress-reduction strategies like yoga, meditation, and breathing exercises (pranayama) to enhance general well-being and immune function. Adequate sleep, regular exercise, and avoidance of dangerous behaviors such as smoking and excessive alcohol use are also necessary.

EXTERNAL TREATMENTS: External treatments in Ayurveda seek to nourish the skin and help its healing process. This may entail the use of herbal pastes, oils, or ointments containing particular herbs and components. Ayurvedic massages and targeted therapies like patra pinda sweda (herbal poultice massage) and lepa (herbal paste application) are widely utilized to increase the therapeutic impact.

It is vital to emphasize that although Ayurvedic techniques may be used as supportive measures in skin cancer care, they should never be regarded as a substitute for standard medical therapies such as surgery, radiation therapy, or chemotherapy. It is necessary to contact a skilled Ayurvedic practitioner and work in concert with a healthcare team to build a complete treatment plan that suits individual requirements and preferences.

Furthermore, it is vital to constantly monitor the course of skin cancer through medical exams, imaging, and testing. Any changes in the condition should be reported to the healthcare professional promptly, and relevant medical measures should be sought without delay.

In summary, Ayurvedic practices may give a comprehensive approach to skin cancer care by concentrating on cleansing, immunological support, and preserving general well-being. However, it is vital to combine Ayurveda with mainstream medical therapies and consult with healthcare specialists for the best effects.

COMBINING CONVENTIONAL AND ALTERNATIVE APPROACHES
SAFETY, REGULATION, AND RESEARCH ON COMPLEMENTARY AND ALTERNATIVE TREATMENTS FOR SKIN CANCER

Combining conventional and alternative treatments in the realm of skin cancer therapy includes merging mainstream medical procedures with complementary and alternative therapies to offer complete care. This approach emphasizes that although traditional therapies like surgery, chemotherapy, and radiation therapy are the norm for controlling skin cancer, alternative treatments may be utilized in combination to optimize results, improve quality of life, and meet individual patient requirements.

Safety is a vital factor when mixing traditional and unconventional procedures. Conventional therapies for skin cancer have undergone significant research, clinical studies, and regulatory approval procedures to show their safety and effectiveness. These therapies are often recommended by medical specialists who follow defined procedures and criteria. However, alternative medicines may lack the same degree of scientific proof, rigorous testing, and regulation.

To guarantee patient safety, it is vital to closely analyze the safety and effectiveness of alternative therapies before combining them with traditional techniques. This may be done by a full grasp of the treatment, evaluating accessible scientific research, engaging with healthcare specialists skilled in both traditional and alternative medicine, and considering patient preferences and values. Open communication and cooperation between healthcare practitioners and patients are crucial to make educated choices about combining therapies.

Regulation of complementary and alternative treatments differs across various nations and areas. Regulatory authorities may have diverse ways to evaluate safety, quality, and effectiveness.

In certain circumstances, alternative medicines may come within the jurisdiction of regulatory bodies responsible for food, nutritional supplements, or natural health goods, rather than particular cancer treatment rules. This regulatory environment underlines the significance of getting information from healthcare experts who are informed about the legal and regulatory frameworks regulating the use of alternative therapies for skin cancer.

Research plays a key role in assessing the efficacy of complementary and alternative therapies for skin cancer. Scientific research, clinical trials, and systematic reviews assist create knowledge on the safety, effectiveness, and possible interactions of alternative medicines with mainstream treatments.

Rigorous studies may also give insight into the mechanisms of action, ideal dose, and possible negative effects of these medicines. It is crucial to highlight that although certain alternative medicines may show promise in the laboratory or early clinical investigations, they may not have sufficient evidence to justify general acceptance as mainstream treatments.

To mix traditional and alternative techniques successfully, multidisciplinary teamwork is crucial. Oncologists, dermatologists, naturopathic physicians, and other healthcare providers should work together to design tailored treatment programs that include both traditional and alternative medicines. This collaborative approach guarantees that patients get the best possible care, including evidence-based therapies while recognizing individual preferences, requirements, and beliefs.

In conclusion, integrating traditional and alternative treatments in the treatment of skin cancer involves careful consideration of safety, regulation, and research. The integration of alternative medicines should be founded on full knowledge of their safety and effectiveness, adherence to regulatory requirements, and evidence-based research.

By participating in multidisciplinary cooperation and open communication with healthcare providers, patients may obtain holistic care that includes the qualities of both traditional and alternative therapies.

QUESTIONS PEOPLE WITH SKIN CANCER CAN ASK THEIR HEALTHCARE PROVIDER ABOUT COMPLEMENTARY AND ALTERNATIVE TREATMENTS

- Are there any complementary or alternative treatments that can be used alongside conventional skin cancer treatments?
- What are the potential benefits of complementary and alternative treatments for skin cancer?
- Are there any risks or side effects associated with these treatments?
- How do complementary and alternative treatments for skin cancer work?
- Can you provide information on the scientific evidence supporting the effectiveness of these treatments?
- What is the recommended dosage or treatment regimen for complementary and alternative treatments?
- Can you suggest any reputable sources or organizations that provide reliable information on these treatments?
- Are there any specific dietary changes or supplements that may be beneficial for skin cancer patients?

- How do these treatments interact with conventional cancer treatments such as surgery, radiation therapy, or chemotherapy?
- Are there any specific complementary or alternative treatments that are known to interfere with conventional treatments?
- Can these treatments help alleviate symptoms such as pain, nausea, or fatigue associated with skin cancer or its treatments?
- Are there any potential drug interactions between these treatments and medications I am currently taking?
- How will these treatments be monitored and evaluated for their effectiveness?
- Can you refer me to a specialist or integrative medicine practitioner who has experience in treating skin cancer patients with complementary and alternative therapies?

- What are the costs associated with these treatments, and will my insurance cover them?
- Can you provide information on any clinical trials or research studies exploring complementary and alternative treatments for skin cancer?
- Are there any specific mind-body techniques, such as meditation or acupuncture, that may be helpful during my treatment?
- Can complementary and alternative treatments help improve my overall well-being and quality of life during the course of my skin cancer treatment?
- What precautions should I take if I decide to pursue complementary or alternative treatments?
- Can you explain the potential mechanisms by which these treatments may exert their effects on skin cancer?

- Are there any specific complementary or alternative treatments that have shown promising results in patients with skin cancer?
- Can these treatments be used as a sole alternative to conventional treatments for skin cancer?
- How do complementary and alternative treatments support the immune system in the context of skin cancer?
- Are there any specific herbal remedies or botanical extracts that have been studied for skin cancer treatment?
- What is the current understanding of the safety and efficacy of these herbal remedies or botanical extracts?
- Can complementary and alternative treatments help prevent the recurrence of skin cancer?
- Are there any potential risks or interactions with these treatments if I have other medical conditions or take other medications?

- Can you provide guidance on finding reliable and evidence-based information about complementary and alternative treatments for skin cancer?
- How do these treatments address the psychological and emotional aspects of skin cancer diagnosis and treatment?
- Are there any specific alternative therapies that can help manage stress and anxiety associated with skin cancer?
- Can complementary and alternative treatments help improve the healing process after surgery or other interventions for skin cancer?
- What are the potential benefits of incorporating mind-body practices such as yoga or tai chi into my treatment plan?
- Are there any complementary or alternative treatments that may help reduce the side effects of conventional

treatments like chemotherapy-induced nausea or radiation-related skin reactions?

- Can you explain the potential risks and benefits of using dietary supplements or vitamins as adjunctive treatments for skin cancer?
- Are there any specific homeopathic remedies that have been explored for skin cancer treatment?
- Can complementary and alternative treatments help manage the fatigue and lack of energy often experienced by skin cancer patients?
- Are there any specific dietary restrictions or recommendations I should follow while undergoing these treatments?
- Can complementary and alternative treatments be used to support the body's detoxification processes during skin cancer treatment?

CHAPTER 5

Foods To Eat and avoid

INTRODUCTION TO SKIN CANCER AND DIET
- Overview of the relevance of nutrition in skin cancer prevention and treatment

Skin cancer is the most frequent kind of cancer globally, and its prevalence is rapidly growing. It generally happens when the skin cells are damaged by the sun's ultraviolet (UV) radiation, resulting in the abnormal proliferation of skin cells. However, additional variables like heredity, exposure to artificial UV sources (e.g., tanning beds), and a weaker immune system may also contribute to its development.

The three primary kinds of skin cancer are basal cell carcinoma (BCC), squamous cell carcinoma (SCC), and melanoma. BCC and SCC are non-melanoma skin cancers that are typically less aggressive than melanoma, which is the worst kind. While early discovery and treatment may lead to favorable results, prevention remains vital.

IMPORTANCE OF DIET IN SKIN CANCER PREVENTION AND MANAGEMENT:
Research has demonstrated that nutrition has a crucial impact on both the prevention and treatment of skin cancer. A healthy and balanced diet may supply critical nutrients and antioxidants that support skin health,

enhance the immune system, and protect against the harmful effects of UV radiation. Here's an outline of the role of nutrition in skin cancer prevention and management:

ANTIOXIDANT PROTECTION:
Certain vitamins and minerals, such as vitamins A, C, E, and selenium, operate as antioxidants in the body. Antioxidants help neutralize damaging free radicals created by UV radiation, reducing oxidative damage to the skin cells. Foods high in antioxidants include colorful fruits and vegetables including berries, citrus fruits, leafy greens, carrots, and bell peppers.

OMEGA-3 FATTY ACIDS:
Omega-3 fatty acids are necessary lipids with significant anti-inflammatory effects. They help decrease inflammation in the body, which is vital for preventing cancer formation and progression. Fatty fish like salmon, mackerel, and sardines are great providers of omega-3 fatty acids.

Plant-based sources include flaxseeds, chia seeds, and walnuts.

CAROTENOIDS:
Carotenoids are plant pigments that give fruits and vegetables their brilliant hues. They work as natural sunscreens, protecting the skin from UV-induced damage. Foods high in carotenoids include tomatoes, sweet potatoes, carrots, spinach, kale, and apricots.

GREEN TEA:
Green tea is a high source of polyphenols, notably epigallocatechin gallate (EGCG), which has been found to exhibit anti-cancer potential. EGCG helps protect the skin from UV radiation-induced damage and may even help limit the formation of skin cancer cells. Incorporating green tea into your diet might bring possible advantages for skin health.

CRUCIFEROUS VEGETABLES:
Cruciferous plants including broccoli, cauliflower, cabbage, and Brussels sprouts

contain chemicals called glucosinolates. These chemicals have been related to a lower risk of different malignancies, including skin cancer. They activate the body's detoxification mechanisms and assist remove potentially hazardous compounds.

HYDRATION:
Staying hydrated is vital for general health, including skin health. Proper hydration helps preserve the skin's moisture barrier, improving its resistance against UV radiation. Drinking a proper quantity of water and ingesting water-rich foods like watermelon, cucumbers, and citrus fruits helps enhance hydration.

SUN-PROTECTIVE NUTRIENTS:
While food alone cannot replace the requirement for sun protection measures like wearing sunscreen and protective clothes, some nutrients may increase the skin's natural resistance against UV radiation. For example, ingesting foods high

in lycopene (tomatoes, watermelon) and polyphenols (berries, dark chocolate) may give some extra sun protection advantages.

CONCLUSION:
It's crucial to highlight that although a good diet may help with skin cancer prevention and treatment, it should be supplemented by other preventative measures. These include avoiding excessive sun exposure, applying sunscreen, wearing protective clothing, and periodically inspecting the skin for any changes or abnormalities. If you have worries about skin cancer or want individualized advice on your food and skin health, it is advisable to speak with a healthcare expert or a qualified dietitian.

THE LINK BETWEEN DIET AND SKIN CANCER RISK
- Identifying dietary variables that enhance the risk of skin cancer

- Exploring the influence of high-fat diets, processed foods, and sugar on skin health

The relationship between nutrition and skin cancer risk has been a focus of scientific inquiry and analysis. While sun exposure and hereditary factors play key roles in the development of skin cancer, new data shows that dietary habits might also impact an individual's vulnerability to this illness. For example, some dietary patterns and components have been related to an elevated risk of skin cancer, including high-fat diets, processed foods, and excessive sugar consumption.

One dietary element that has been associated with skin cancer risk is the intake of high-fat meals. Research has revealed that diets heavy in saturated fats and trans fats might lead to inflammation and oxidative stress, both of which are known to increase the development of cancer. These kinds of fats are typically found in meals such as red meat, butter, margarine, and processed snacks.

Processed meals, which are often heavy in refined carbs, bad fats, and artificial additives, have also been related to an increased risk of skin cancer. These meals frequently lack vital nutrients and are linked with a higher glycemic index, leading to fast rises in blood sugar levels. Studies have revealed that high glycemic index meals might induce insulin resistance and inflammation, variables that may lead to skin cancer development.

Excessive sugar consumption has emerged as another dietary component that may impact skin health and skin cancer risk. Consuming significant quantities of sugar may contribute to chronic inflammation, weight gain, and metabolic abnormalities. Additionally, increased sugar consumption may lead to the formation of advanced glycation end products (AGEs), which can damage collagen and elastin fibers in the skin and hasten skin aging.

While the direct relationship between sugar intake and skin cancer is still being explored, the harmful effect of excessive sugar consumption on general health raises worries over its possible involvement in skin cancer development.

Furthermore, several studies have revealed that diets low in particular nutrients may potentially raise the risk of skin cancer. For example, poor consumption of antioxidants, such as vitamins A, C, and E, may hamper the body's capacity to neutralize damaging free radicals and defend against UV-induced damage. Similarly, deficits in omega-3 fatty acids, usually found in fatty fish, walnuts, and flaxseeds, have been related to an increased risk of skin cancer owing to their anti-inflammatory characteristics.

It is crucial to highlight that although these dietary habits have been associated with an increased risk of skin cancer, they are not the primary drivers of the illness.

Other variables, such as genetics, sun exposure, and individual sensitivity, also play key roles in the development of skin cancer. However, adopting a balanced diet that includes a range of nutrient-rich foods, such as fruits, vegetables, whole grains, lean proteins, and healthy fats, may improve general skin health and perhaps minimize the risk of skin cancer.

In conclusion, while more study is required to completely understand the complicated interaction between food and skin cancer risk, existing data shows that particular dietary patterns and components might alter an individual's vulnerability to this illness. High-fat diets, processed foods, and excessive sugar consumption have been related to an increased risk of skin cancer, possibly owing to their effect on inflammation, oxidative stress, insulin resistance, and nutritional deficiencies. Therefore, adopting a balanced and nutrient-rich diet is vital for keeping good skin and perhaps minimizing the incidence of skin cancer.

PROTECTIVE FOODS FOR SKIN CANCER PREVENTION
- The efficacy of fruits and vegetables in lowering skin cancer risk
- Superfoods and their potential advantages for skin health

PROTECTIVE FOODS FOR SKIN CANCER PREVENTION
Skin cancer is one of the most frequent kinds of cancer globally. While there are several risk factors connected with its development, such as exposure to UV radiation, genetics, and certain medical conditions, adopting a balanced diet may play a vital part in avoiding skin cancer. For

example, integrating preventive foods, such as fruits and vegetables, into your diet may give major advantages for skin health and minimize the risk of skin cancer.

THE POWER OF FRUITS AND VEGETABLES IN REDUCING SKIN CANCER RISK:

ANTIOXIDANT PROTECTION: Fruits and vegetables are rich in antioxidants, which help battle oxidative stress generated by free radicals in the body. Free radicals may harm cells, including skin cells, and contribute to the development of skin cancer. Antioxidants, such as vitamins C and E, carotenoids (e.g., beta-carotene), and flavonoids, can neutralize these dangerous free radicals, hence lowering the risk of skin cancer.

SUN PROTECTION: Some fruits and vegetables have natural ingredients that give sun protection from the inside. For example, some foods including citrus fruits, strawberries, and kiwis are rich in vitamin C, which has been demonstrated to help protect the skin from UV-induced damage.

Additionally, crops like leafy greens and cruciferous vegetables include chemicals called sulforaphane and indole-3-carbinol, respectively, which may have protective properties against UV radiation.

ANTI-INFLAMMATORY EFFECTS: Chronic inflammation in the body may lead to several disorders, including skin cancer. Fruits and vegetables are recognized for their anti-inflammatory qualities owing to their high abundance of phytochemicals and fiber. By lowering inflammation, these foods may help promote healthy skin and minimize the risk of skin cancer.

SUPERFOODS AND THEIR POTENTIAL BENEFITS FOR SKIN HEALTH:

BERRIES: Berries, such as blueberries, strawberries, and raspberries, are filled with antioxidants and phytochemicals, including anthocyanins and vitamin C. These chemicals have been related to decreased DNA damage produced by UV radiation and may help prevent the development of skin cancer. Including a variety of berries in your diet may offer a strong boost to your skin health.

TOMATOES: Tomatoes are rich in a chemical called lycopene, which gives them their red color. Lycopene is a strong antioxidant that has been associated with a decreased risk of numerous forms of cancer, including skin cancer. Consuming cooked or processed tomatoes, such as tomato sauce or paste, boosts the availability of lycopene for the body.

LEAFY GREENS: Dark leafy greens, such as spinach, kale, and Swiss chard, are good sources of vitamins A, C, and E, as well as other antioxidants. These nutrients help protect the skin from UV-induced damage and support overall skin health. Including leafy greens in your diet may give crucial vitamins and minerals for skin cancer prevention.

CRUCIFEROUS VEGETABLES: Vegetables including broccoli, cauliflower, cabbage, and Brussels sprouts belong to the cruciferous family. They contain several phytochemicals, including sulforaphane and indole-3-carbinol, which have demonstrated potential anti-cancer benefits. These chemicals may help protect the skin from UV radiation and perhaps prevent skin cancer.

CITRUS FRUITS: Citrus fruits, such as oranges, lemons, and grapefruits, are high in vitamin C and other antioxidants. Vitamin C promotes collagen formation, which helps preserve the flexibility and health of the skin. Additionally, citrus fruits' antioxidant content may help lessen the oxidative damage produced by UV radiation, thereby lowering the risk of skin cancer.

It's crucial to remember that although ingesting preventive foods may help lower the incidence of skin cancer, they should not be seen as a substitute for proper therapy.

THE ROLE OF CAROTENOIDS IN SKIN CANCER PREVENTION
- Exploring the preventive benefits of carotenoids on skin health
- Foods rich in carotenoids and their potential advantages

Carotenoids are a family of naturally occurring pigments found in numerous fruits and vegetables. They are responsible for the brilliant hues observed in foods like carrots, tomatoes, peppers, and leafy greens. Carotenoids have been widely investigated for their multiple health advantages, including their involvement in skin cancer prevention.

Skin cancer is a serious public health problem globally, with overexposure to ultraviolet (UV) radiation being the leading risk factor. UV exposure may generate oxidative stress and DNA damage, leading to the development of skin cancer. However, carotenoids exhibit various qualities that make them excellent antioxidants and photoprotective agents, hence lowering the risk of skin cancer.

One of the major methods via which carotenoids exert their protective benefits is by acting as antioxidants. They have the potential to neutralize damaging free radicals created by UV light and other environmental conditions. Free radicals are extremely reactive chemicals that may damage biological components, including DNA, proteins, and lipids. By scavenging these free radicals, carotenoids help prevent oxidative damage to skin cells and lower the risk of skin cancer.

Moreover, carotenoids also exhibit anti-inflammatory effects. UV radiation induces an inflammatory reaction in the skin, which may lead to skin damage and cancer formation. Carotenoids have been demonstrated to influence the inflammatory response by decreasing the formation of pro-inflammatory chemicals. This anti-inflammatory impact helps minimize the damaging effects of UV radiation on the skin.

Another essential element of carotenoids in skin cancer prevention is their involvement in photoprotection. These pigments are known to absorb UV light, especially in the UVA and UVB spectrum, and disperse the absorbed energy as heat. By doing so, carotenoids inhibit the penetration of UV radiation into the deeper layers of the skin, so decreasing the damage caused by UV exposure.

It's worth mentioning that various forms of carotenoids may have variable degrees of photoprotective properties. Some of the most well-studied carotenoids are beta-carotene, lycopene, lutein, and zeaxanthin. Beta-carotene, present in carrots, sweet potatoes, and spinach, is turned into vitamin A in the body and has been related to lower skin cancer risk. Lycopene, abundant in tomatoes, watermelon, and pink grapefruit, has been demonstrated to protect against UV-induced skin damage. Lutein and zeaxanthin, contained in dark leafy greens, broccoli, and peas, have also been associated to decrease skin cancer risk.

Incorporating carotenoid-rich foods into your diet may offer a natural source of photoprotection for your skin. Consuming a range of fruits and vegetables, especially those with strong colors, guarantees a diversified intake of carotenoids. Aim for a kaleidoscope of colors on your plate to optimize the advantages. Additionally, it's crucial to remember that carotenoids are fat-soluble, so ingesting them alongside a source of healthy fats, such as olive oil or avocado, might boost their absorption.

While carotenoids play a key role in skin cancer prevention, it's essential to remember that they are only one component of a total sun protection plan. It is still necessary to adopt other sun safety precautions, such as wearing protective clothing, applying broad-spectrum sunscreen, finding cover during peak solar hours, and avoiding excessive sun exposure.

In conclusion, carotenoids have considerable preventive benefits against skin cancer via their antioxidant, anti-inflammatory, and photoprotective capabilities. Including a range of carotenoid-rich foods in your diet may improve skin health and give an extra layer of protection against the detrimental effects of UV radiation. However, it's vital to complement this dietary strategy with additional sun protection strategies for total skin cancer prevention.

ANTI-INFLAMMATORY DIET FOR SKIN CANCER MANAGEMENT
- Understanding the role of inflammation in skin cancer progression
- Dietary recommendations to minimize inflammation and promote skin health

UNDERSTANDING THE ROLE OF INFLAMMATION IN SKIN CANCER PROGRESSION:
Inflammation has a key role in the development and progression of several illnesses, including cancer. In the case of skin cancer, persistent inflammation may

contribute to the start, development, and advancement of cancer cells. Inflammatory processes in the skin may be caused by many causes such as ultraviolet (UV) radiation, environmental pollutants, and certain lifestyle variables.

Chronic inflammation may lead to DNA damage, poor immunological function, and an imbalance of pro-inflammatory and anti-inflammatory chemicals in the body. These elements produce an environment that favors the development and survival of cancer cells. Therefore, adopting an anti-inflammatory diet may be a useful method to control skin cancer by lowering inflammation and increasing overall skin health.

DIETARY STRATEGIES TO REDUCE INFLAMMATION AND SUPPORT SKIN HEALTH:
INCREASE ANTIOXIDANT INTAKE: Antioxidants help neutralize free radicals,

which are highly reactive chemicals that may harm cells and lead to inflammation. Include a range of fruits and vegetables high in antioxidants, such as berries, leafy greens, carrots, and tomatoes, in your diet.

OMEGA-3 FATTY ACIDS: Omega-3 fatty acids have significant anti-inflammatory capabilities and may help control immunological responses. Include foods rich in omega-3s, such as fatty fish (salmon, mackerel, sardines), chia seeds, flaxseeds, and walnuts.

LIMIT OMEGA-6 FATTY ACIDS: While omega-3s are good, excessive consumption of omega-6 fatty acids, found in vegetable oils (soybean, maize, sunflower), might increase inflammation. Reduce the intake of processed and fried meals that commonly include these oils.

CHOOSE HEALTHY FATS: Opt for healthier fats, such as olive oil, avocados, and almonds, which include monounsaturated fats. These fats have anti-inflammatory qualities and supply the necessary elements for skin health.

COLORFUL PLANT FOODS: Include a variety of colorful fruits and vegetables in your diet. They are rich in phytochemicals, vitamins, and minerals that boost immune function and decrease inflammation.

FIBER-RICH MEALS: Consuming high-fiber meals including whole grains, legumes, and vegetables may help maintain a healthy gut flora. A healthy gut microbiota is vital for controlling inflammation and promoting general health.

SPICES AND HERBS: Turmeric, ginger, garlic, and green tea are recognized for their anti-inflammatory qualities. Incorporate these spices and herbs into your meals to improve taste and give possible anti-inflammatory effects.

STAY HYDRATED: Drinking a sufficient quantity of water is vital for maintaining skin hydration and general health. It helps flush out pollutants and promotes proper cellular function.

LIMIT ADDED SUGARS: High consumption of added sugars might increase inflammation. Reduce your intake of sugary drinks, processed foods, and desserts.

LIMIT PROCESSED FOODS: Processed foods frequently include high quantities of harmful fats, added sugars, and artificial additives. Opt for full, unprocessed foods as much as possible.

It's crucial to remember that although an anti-inflammatory diet might be useful, it should be supplemented with other medical treatments and tactics indicated by healthcare specialists for controlling skin cancer. Consult with your healthcare physician or a qualified dietician for individualized advice and assistance suited to your unique requirements and condition.

FOODS TO AVOID

As a skin cancer patient, it is crucial to pay close attention to your food and make educated decisions that may support your general health and assist in your recovery. While there are no particular foods that directly cause or cure skin cancer, some dietary choices may help lower the chance of recurrence or improve skin health. On the other hand, there are certain foods you may wish to avoid or take in moderation to support your therapy and prevent possible consequences.

PROCESSED MEATS: Foods like bacon, sausage, hot dogs, and deli meats are generally rich in nitrates, preservatives, and additives that may be damaging to your health. Studies have connected the intake of processed meats to an elevated risk of some malignancies. Opt for lean, unprocessed meats or plant-based protein sources instead.

SUGARY AND REFINED FOODS: Foods that are heavy in added sugars, such as sugary drinks, sweets, cakes, and cookies, might contribute to inflammation and possibly damage your immune system. High consumption of refined carbs, including white bread and spaghetti, may also affect your blood sugar levels. Instead, pick whole grains, fresh fruits, and natural sweeteners like honey or maple syrup in moderation.

TRANS FATS: Trans fats are artificially manufactured fats present in many processed and fried meals, including fast food, packaged snacks, and commercially baked items. These fats lead to inflammation and may badly influence your heart health. Opt for healthy fats like olive oil, avocados, and almonds.

EXCESSIVE ALCOHOL: Alcohol might damage your immune system and make it more difficult for your body to recover from skin cancer or its treatment. Excessive alcohol use is also related to an elevated risk of some malignancies. If you do want to drink, do it in moderation and select healthier alternatives like red wine, which includes antioxidants.

HIGH-GLYCEMIC FOODS: Foods having a high glycemic index, such as white rice, potatoes, and sugary cereals, may induce a quick jump in blood sugar levels. This may lead to increased inflammation and possibly disturbances in insulin levels. Opt for low-glycemic options like quinoa, sweet potatoes, and whole grains, which are metabolized more slowly.

EXCESSIVE SODIUM: Foods heavy in sodium, such as processed snacks, canned soups, and fast food, may induce water retention and may lead to hypertension.

Limiting your salt consumption may assist maintain a healthy blood pressure and general well-being. Opt for fresh, handmade foods seasoned with herbs and spices instead.

Remember that although avoiding some foods is vital, focusing on a balanced and diverse diet is also critical. Prioritize entire, nutrient-dense foods including fruits, vegetables, lean meats, and healthy fats. Consult with your healthcare team or a qualified dietitian to build a specific nutrition plan that best meets your requirements and supports your skin cancer therapy.

CREATING A SKIN-HEALTHY DIET PLAN
- Practical advice for establishing a food plan focusing on skin cancer prevention and management

- Sample meal ideas and recipes for enhancing skin health

Creating a skin-healthy food plan may play a vital part in preserving healthy skin, avoiding skin cancer, and treating other skin diseases. By including specific nutrients, antioxidants, and healthy fats into your diet, you can promote your skin's health and general well-being. Here are some practical guidelines for establishing a food plan focusing on skin health and example meal ideas and recipes to achieve a bright complexion.

INCLUDE ANTIOXIDANT-RICH FOODS:
Antioxidants help protect the skin from damage produced by free radicals, which may lead to premature aging and skin cancer. Include a variety of colorful fruits and vegetables in your diet, since they are high in antioxidants. Berries, spinach, kale, carrots, bell peppers, and tomatoes are

wonderful alternatives. You may eat them in salads, smoothies, stir-fries, or as snacks.

SAMPLE MEAL IDEA: Spinach and Berry Salad

INGREDIENTS:
- 2 cups fresh spinach leaves
- 1 cup mixed berries (strawberries, blueberries, raspberries)
- 1/4 cup walnuts
- 2 tablespoons feta cheese (optional)
- Balsamic vinaigrette dressing (to taste)

INSTRUCTIONS:
- Wash and dry the spinach leaves.
- In a bowl, add spinach, mixed berries, walnuts, and feta cheese.
- Drizzle with balsamic vinaigrette dressing and toss lightly to coat.
- Serve as a side dish or add grilled chicken for a full supper.

INCORPORATE HEALTHY FATS:

Healthy fats, such as omega-3 fatty acids, are vital for preserving skin health and lowering inflammation. Include sources of omega-3s in your diet, such as fatty fish (salmon, mackerel, sardines), flaxseeds, chia seeds, and walnuts. These fats help keep the skin hydrated and may reduce symptoms of inflammatory skin diseases including eczema and psoriasis.

SAMPLE MEAL IDEA: Grilled Salmon with Quinoa and Steamed Vegetables

INGREDIENTS:
- 1 salmon fillet
- 1 tablespoon olive oil
- Salt and pepper to taste
- 1/2 cup cooked quinoa
- Steamed veggies (broccoli, carrots, asparagus)

INSTRUCTIONS:

- Preheat the grill.
- Rub the salmon fillet with olive oil and season with salt and pepper.
- Grill the salmon for approximately 5-7 minutes each side or until cooked through.
- Serve the grilled salmon with a dish of cooked quinoa and steamed veggies.

STAY HYDRATED:

Proper hydration is vital for keeping healthy skin. Drink a proper quantity of water throughout the day to keep your skin moisturized and maintain a healthy complexion. Additionally, incorporate hydrating items in your diet, such as melons, cucumbers, oranges, and leafy greens.

SAMPLE MEAL IDEA: Cucumber and Watermelon Salad

INGREDIENTS:

- 2 cups diced watermelon
- 1 cucumber, peeled and sliced
- 1/4 red onion, thinly sliced
- 2 teaspoons fresh mint leaves, chopped
- 1 tablespoon lime juice
- Salt and pepper to taste

INSTRUCTIONS:
- In a large bowl, mix watermelon, cucumber, red onion, and mint leaves.
- Drizzle with lime juice and season with salt and pepper.
- Toss lightly to mix.
- Serve chilled as a pleasant side dish.

LIMIT PROCESSED FOODS AND ADDED SUGARS: Processed foods and foods rich in added sugars may lead to inflammation and oxidative stress, which can adversely affect the skin. Opt for healthy meals and reduce your use of sugary snacks, drinks, and processed munchies.

HYDRATION:
Maintaining proper moisture is vital for good skin. Drink lots of water throughout the day to keep your skin moisturized and encourage detoxification. Herbal teas and infused water with cucumber, lemon, or mint may also be pleasant and hydrating choices.

SAMPLE MEAL IDEA:
BREAKFAST: Green smoothie composed of spinach, cucumber, banana, and coconut water.
LUNCH: Vegetable soup with healthy grain crackers and a side of herbal tea.
SNACK: Infused water with chopped lemon and mint.
DINNER: Grilled shrimp skewers with a side of steamed broccoli and a glass of water.

VITAMINS AND MINERALS:
Ensure an appropriate diet of key vitamins and minerals for good skin. Vitamin C

assists in collagen formation and wound healing, while vitamin E gives protection against UV damage. Zinc is crucial for skin regeneration and helps the immune system. Include foods like citrus fruits, nuts and seeds, whole grains, and legumes to satisfy these nutritional demands.

SAMPLE MEAL IDEA:
BREAKFAST: Whole grain bread topped with avocado, sliced tomatoes, and a sprinkling of pumpkin seeds.
LUNCH: Quinoa salad with roasted veggies (bell peppers, zucchini, and eggplant), chickpeas, and a lemon-tahini dressing.
SNACK: Orange slices and a handful of almonds.
DINNER: Grilled chicken breast with sautéed spinach and brown rice.

OMEGA-3 FATTY ACIDS:
Incorporate foods high in omega-3 fatty acids into your diet. Omega-3 fatty acids contain anti-inflammatory characteristics,

which may help regulate skin irritation and enhance skin health. Good sources of omega-3s include fatty fish (salmon, mackerel, sardines), walnuts, chia seeds, and flaxseeds.

SAMPLE MEAL IDEA:
BREAKFAST: Overnight oats cooked with almond milk, chia seeds, and topped with crushed walnuts and sliced bananas.
LUNCH: Grilled salmon salad with mixed greens, cherry tomatoes, cucumbers, and a sprinkle of olive oil and balsamic vinegar.
SNACK: A handful of walnuts and a slice of fruit.
DINNER: Baked trout with steamed broccoli and quinoa.